MW00873924

Rebuilding Your Temple

Blueprints for True and Lasting Health

By Stacy Mal

Certified Health Coach
Blogger/Author
Media Executive
Plexus Worldwide Ambassador

Gray Matter Media, Inc.
North East, PA USA
www.GrayMatterMediaInc.com

Copyright

Rebuilding Your Temple: Blueprints for True and Lasting Health

By Stacy Mal

Cover Design: Gray Matter Media, Inc.
Cover Photo: Tabitha Bowman

Published by Gray Matter Media, Inc.
P.O. Box 227
North East, PA 16428
www.GrayMatterMedia.com

© 2019 by Gray Matter Media, Inc.

ISBN # 9781695834026

In loving memory of my grandfather,

Frank Anthony Knight II

Table of Contents

Introduction

The Bible says that when God made man and woman, He gave them dominion over every living thing and every plant yielding seed... and that everything was "very good." (Gen. 1:27-31) Through this, we see a glimpse of God's original (and very natural) plan for our physical health. Adam and Eve lived in a luscious garden, surrounded by full rivers. There was no pollution, disease, or want.

Granted, the sin of Adam and Eve changed all that, and they were forever banned from that "good" garden. In fact, humanity became _so_ tainted that God later sent a catastrophic flood to cleanse the earth, renew His creation, and rebuild His people. We can hear his intention as He calls Noah out of the ark. "Everything that lives and moves about will be food for you," God said. "Just as I gave you the green plants, I now give you everything." (Gen. 9:3)

Once again, God stepped in, and things were "good" again.

Fast forward to today. Today, we see that humans have misused their dominion by raising animals (i.e., living things) in poor conditions, then giving them antibiotics and hormones that are harmful to human health. Today, we see plant yielding seeds that have been biochemically altered or genetically modified to withstand copious amounts of pesticides, also harmful to human health. We see the plants themselves are deconstructed, processed, treated, bleached, and refined. We see that soil is overused and devoid of nutrients. We see that much of our food no longer comes from the earth that God made, but from a factory that man-made.

Not surprisingly, things are not very "good" anymore. Even if you are not Christian and do not give credence to the Bible, I think we can agree that America is experiencing a major health decline.

Almost 40% of U.S. adults are now classified as obese. (1) More than 90 million Americans have been diagnosed with Cardiovascular Disease. (2) Nearly 40% of men and women will be diagnosed with cancer at some point during their lifetimes. (3) Approximately 50 million Americans (20% of the population, or one in five people) suffer from one or more of the now 80 classified autoimmune diseases. (4) More than 100 million U.S. adults are now living with diabetes or prediabetes. (5) And nearly 70% of Americans are taking at least one prescription drug (and more than half of the population is taking two). (6)

I don't believe this is what God planned for us. By altering our food in such drastic ways, I believe we got off track. We moved away from His original plan as it relates to nutrition, and we are now suffering the effects of this derailment. We are like runaway steam engines going downhill. We are racing faster and faster toward the end of our days, as life expectancy declines year after year, despite advances in modern medicine.

But, friend, God is trying to step in once again. He is calling us back to the plan.

It is for this reason that I have written this book. Because, despite the statistics, we are *not* doomed. And despite all the conflicting information thrown at us (eat this, don't eat that), it's not as complicated as it sounds. To get back on track toward wellness, I believe we simply need to go back to the basics, back to the way *God* originally intended it to be. And we need to listen to our bodies.

As a Christian, I believe that God is the Architect and the original Builder of the temple of the body. I believe as part of His creation our bodies are "good." However, like any physical structure, the "elements" can wear on it over time. The temple can suffer damage as well as progressive, age-related erosion and decay.

When this happens, we can either address it or keep coasting like a steam engine. How do we address it? Well, we can make a couple of quick fixes (things that will help us "get by" just a little while longer). Or, we can look at the underlying damage and decay, where it came from, and try to rebuild. For example, if you are suffering from fatigue, you could make a "quick fix" by either drinking more coffee or more energy drinks. Or, you could work with your doctor to find out the cause of the fatigue.

The two choices are *drastically* different approaches. Quick fixes often just mask symptoms. It's like slapping a coat of paint on mold-infested walls. It looks like you've fixed it, but you've just covered it up for a time.

Deciding to rebuild, on the other hand, involves so much more—killing the mold, probably replacing boards and insulation, and *then* repainting. It also involves looking at other areas of the house that may have contributed to the mold—be it a plumbing leak, a faulty roof, or a weak foundation, etc. My point is: *rebuilding* is all-encompassing.

Such is the case here, too. Rebuilding the temple of the body is all-encompassing. Instead of doing little things to address *symptoms* (like taking more ibuprofen for pain) rebuilding encourages a "whole body" approach (like trying to reduce inflammation—and thereby pain— with better food choices).

The Blueprint

I have compiled the information in this book through years of study, research, and prayer, and I believe this material outlines the plan of the original Architect and Creator of the temple—who, by the way, predates diabetes, autoimmune disease, and cancer. Put simply; I believe this book is God's blueprint for the human body. As a health coach, author, and media executive, I am merely a "secretary" who has re-drawn the design for you.

Therefore, please understand: this book is not, *NOT* intended to serve as medical advice, or to replace it in any way. No, this book is for educational purposes only. This information is meant to be discussed with your doctor, who should serve as the general contractor throughout your rebuilding project. It is your *doctor* who will need to give you the go-ahead, approve every phase, and call all the shots. As I said, I am merely the secretary in this case. I am not your contractor or your doctor.

The purpose of this book is to start a conversation between you and your practitioner, to help the two of you begin the rebuilding process *together*. I cannot stress this enough. It is imperative that you work closely with your doctor during every single phase of this rebuild, especially if you have a preexisting condition or are taking any medication.

And notice I said work "with" your doctor. Your doctor is the contractor which means he/she will guide you and oversee your progress, but your doctor will not *do* the building for you. That job, my friend, belongs to you. YOU are the one who is going to have to put in the effort. You are the one who is going to have to dig deep, make sacrifices, and work hard at this. You and only you. It's your temple, and no one is going to rebuild it for you.

It's also important to note that blueprints are merely a starting point for any building project. Often, blueprints need to be tweaked along the way. Unexpected things can pop up—especially when it comes to renovations. There can be hidden damage or areas that were never built to code, and these things will likely require a reevaluation and an adjustment to the plan.

It's the same when rebuilding your temple. Yes, there is a standard blueprint for the human body—which might work "as is" for a lot of people—but *not* everyone. Some "temples" have been damaged... maybe from years of eating poorly, toxin exposure, or stress. Other temples were not hereditarily "built to code" originally, in one area or another... maybe they inherited food allergies, genetic mutations, or dysbiosis during delivery.

My point is, the blueprint is a starting point that may need to be tweaked as you go. What works for one person, might not work for you. While we are all human beings, we are vastly and immeasurably different ones—with different genetics, predispositions, environments, preexisting conditions, ages, sexes, stress levels, toxin exposures, etcetera, etcetera, etcetera. That means that the vague (and often misused) term "eating healthy" can mean many different things to many different people.

For example, the vegetarian diet might be healthy for many, but for someone with mental health issues, vitamin B12 deficiency, and an MTHFR genetic mutation, it could be disastrous. The ketogenic diet also might be very healthy for many, but for a lean woman with adrenal fatigue undergoing intense training, it could be disastrous.

Just because someone found the diet that's right for them, does not mean it's "the" diet for everyone. Even if your bestie lost 60 pounds doing something that sounds healthy, doesn't mean it's the healthiest thing for you personally. Unfortunately, many people do not understand this—especially on social media, where everyone seems to know everything—and the results of "generalizing" can be tragic.

Take this scenario for example. A newly converted vegan is pressuring her struggling friend to go vegan. Her friend has ADHD, thyroid dysfunction, and other health issues that need ample protein, which is sometimes difficult to get on a vegan diet. Regardless, the friend goes vegan anyway and her health declines. She feels horrible. What's worse, she now feels like a failure and gives up on her health altogether. She feels like she is unfixable.

Or take this scenario: Someone is on social media bashing the ketogenic diet (because it didn't work for them). Unknowingly this person scares away many friends with insulin resistance who may have experienced a magical sort of health transformation via that strategy. Their friends then continue to eat carbs, while struggling with carb addiction, fatigue, and high blood sugar. Over time, they too, begin to feel unfixable, and they give up.

Please understand that healthy eating is not "one-size-fits-all." The blueprint is not carved in stone. Sure, there are fundamental basics, yes. But the details can vary dramatically. And that's precisely why this book was written. It was written to help you discover *your* blueprint, the diet, and lifestyle that best fits your unique temple.

So, as you read through each chapter, I encourage you to take notes, underline, and highlight information that specifically pertains to _you_ and your unique needs. Record this information in the *Rebuilding Your Temple Workbook for Individual and*

Group Study and discuss it with your doctor. Chapter by chapter you will start to develop the plan that is right for you.

Supplements and Patience

As you will see, I talk a lot about products in this book. But remember: all supplements must be approved by your doctor first. Supplements can be very beneficial, yes. I'm a big fan of them, personally. But they can also be dangerous if not taken properly. Again, what works for one person, might not work for everyone. Only your practitioner (your general contractor) can make that call for you.

Also, even if your doctor approves some supplements, it's important to understand that they won't rebuild your temple for you either. A supplement (no matter how good it is) is not going to magically "fix" you. Supplements are merely _tools_ to help you rebuild. A hammer won't build a house by itself, but it sure can make the job easier than pounding a nail with a rock or your fist. The same is true with the supplements that I will reference throughout this book.

These supplements are what I believe to be some of the highest quality products on the market—many with patented, tested, and proven ingredients, unmatched by other brands. They are the "cream of the crop," so to speak, in my opinion. Plexus Worldwide® (the brand I have chosen to use as my personal "temple tools") offers a wide variety of supplements that can be beneficial on multiple body systems. But, even still, these must be used correctly, with patience, and the right materials for them to be of any benefit.

The best drill or the most-powerful nail gun on the market won't erase the fact that you're using warped or rotten boards and curved, rusty nails. The same is true when rebuilding your temple. Taking high-quality supplements won't erase the fact that you're eating trans fat and harmful chemicals in your processed food. At best, you might slow further damage, temporarily, but you're not really "rebuilding."

To *rebuild*, you must work with quality *materials* too. In other words, you must eat quality food. Supplements are the tools; foods are the materials. These two things go hand-in-hand. You do not want to use quality materials without any tools, and you do not want to use the best tools with junky materials. _Both_ are of great importance in any rebuild. But, even still, they do not guarantee a fix any more than a nail gun and a sheet of plywood guarantee a house. You, friend, need to work hard, and you need a professional.

To do it right—to rebuild properly—will take time, diligence, patience and perseverance. You also must do it in phases, working on one thing at a time. A contractor doesn't have people pouring a concrete foundation at the same time builders are trying to frame walls. You don't have the drywallers finish walls before the electricians run wire either. Rebuilding a home needs to be done strategically, in phases—and so does rebuilding your temple. You simply cannot do everything all at the same time.

So, I do not recommend reading this book quickly. Do not devour it overnight, and then try to implement everything in it all at once. In my opinion, that's a surefire way to get overwhelmed and quit. This book was not written with that pace in mind. So, please, take your time with each phase and each project. Read the chapters carefully, taking notes. Learn _how_ to do the job, and then implement the information.

On the other hand, some of you won't want to devour this book. Some of you will be tempted to skim and skip chapters. You will assume that some chapters do not pertain to you after you read the title or the first couple of paragraphs. You may look at the keto chapter and think _"I'm never doing that"_ and so you will want to skip it. Or, maybe you already follow a ketogenic diet so you will want to skip the chapter on carbs and bread.

Either way, please do not skip any chapters. There are important points in each one that will benefit you. Even if you don't eat bread and carbs, you won't want to miss other crucial parts in the chapter... for example, those on autoimmune disease. Even if you know you will never cut carbs and go keto, you won't want to miss the other parts in that chapter... like the importance of insulin and how blood sugars actually work. Remember, to do it _right_ takes time and patience. You can't achieve success by cutting corners.

The Workbook

As I mentioned before, there is a supplemental book called _The Rebuilding Your Temple Workbook for Individual and Group Study_ that I strongly advise purchasing. It is a vital companion that provides chapter recaps, easy to find charts, product dosing schedules, and places for you to take personal notes, which can serve as discussion points for you and your doctor.

This is important because there is an enormous amount of information that is presented in this book. The workbook will serve as a sort of strainer, sifting through the material that is most relevant for you personally. Your notes can then serve as a quick reference for you, for many years to come.

The workbook also serves as a group study that provides discussion questions, challenges, even optional scripture passages for every phase (for those who are interested in staying close to the Architect as they rebuild.) Doing this with a group of friends or family members is _highly_ recommended. The group format not only makes the rebuild more fun and engaging; it also provides you with a network of support when things get difficult. And they _will_ get difficult. A group holds you accountable, too, so you will be more likely to stick with it to the very end.

If you would like to do this in a group format, but you are not sure how to go about it, consider purchasing _The Rebuilding Your Temple Group Leader Guide._ This is a step-by-step guidebook that not only helps you start a group (online or in person), but it also helps you navigate through each of the meetings as a leader or facilitator. You never have to come up with your own material or prepare for the meetings. Everything you need is right there. It even provides you with flyers to advertise the group before it starts and things to post for each phase.

No matter which way you decide to implement this protocol (alone or in a group format) the most important thing to remember is to take your time with each phase and see it through to the end. For those of you who are doing this primarily for weight loss, you may be tempted to stop reading once you decide on a diet, or once the weight starts to come off. I advise you _not_ to do that if you want the weight to _stay_ off. Keep going to the end. But make sure you understand the information from each section and make sure you are comfortable with it, before proceeding.

For some of you, this will be so foreign to you that it will be like adopting a whole new lifestyle, phase by phase. Don't let that discourage you. Be optimistic, excited, and patient. Remember: it's more important to do this correctly than to do it quickly. If that means you have to spend two weeks or even two months on one phase, then so be it. As long as when you move on to the next phase, you feel confident about the work you put into the last phase.

The Most Important Rebuild You'll Ever Do

This strategy is a whole-body lifestyle pulled together from a collection of sources, studies, and prayer. This is "rebuilding," friend, which takes time. You can't rebuild your house overnight, and you can't rebuild your temple overnight either.

Unfortunately, I've coached MANY impatient clients who don't understand that. They want to be healthy yesterday or skinny by next Tuesday—even though they've been unhealthy or overweight for 15, 20, or 40 years. Friend, that's not how it works. That's not how _anything_ works. Real, lasting change takes work, and work takes time.

Think about it: some people will spend tedious months or _years_ building their dream home. They devote that time to it because it's important to them. They want to live their whole life in that house. They want it to last and withstand the elements for many years to come. They want to live life and accomplish their dreams in that house. They want to be comfortable and happy there. They want to raise a family there, entertain friends there. They want to pass on that house to future generations as a legacy.

How much more important is the temple of your body? A body that embraces friends and serves family, and (if you are in the child-bearing years) passes on temple genetics as a legacy to future generations. A body that's home to not only you but to the Spirit of God who dwells in you. A body that is called according to a purpose, to accomplish a mission, to affect some _good_ and everlasting change in this world. A body that is meant to lead, guide, teach, or protect others.

Isn't it important that your temple is strong enough to also withstand the elements for many years to come? Quite frankly, you can always get a new house. But you only get one temple (one body) to last your entire lifetime. So, in my opinion, there is not a more important "rebuild" than this one (except maybe the rebuilding of your soul, which I've written about in the book _Rebuilding Your Temple Garden_, available Fall 2019 on Amazon.com.)

So, friends, please understand the scope of the work that is involved in this, and do not take it lightly. If you are not quite ready to embark on something so grand and in-depth—if you are not ready to completely rebuild your temple yet—then maybe this book isn't for you, _right now_. Maybe you need to build yourself up mentally and emotionally first. And that's ok. That's perfectly ok. But don't put it off for too long. It's amazing how fast a steam engine can coast downhill... and how fast a temple can reach a state of disease.

A Fellow Builder

I know I said I was the secretary here, but I would be remiss if I did not tell you I am also a fellow builder. I have implemented this protocol in my own life because I once was a temple in ruins, quite literally falling down. It started early on in my life and spiraled out of control.

I had my first anxiety attack at age 6.
I had my first taste of depression at 12.

I had my first visit to a cardiologist at 13.
I had my first ambulance ride at 14.
I took my first cardiac medication at 14 too.
I had my first heart procedure at 15.
I had my second heart procedure at 16.
I had my third heart procedure at 17.
I first suspected I had ADD at 18.
I was prescribed my first hormone medication at 19.
I saw my first endocrinologist at 20.
I got my first glucose monitor at 21.
I had my fourth heart procedure at 22.
I had my first vascular diagnosis at 23.
I was taking 20 pills a day (all prescriptions) at 24.
I was diagnosed with dysautonomia at 24 also.
I was 120 pounds overweight at 25.
I started having severe numbness at 26.
I saw my first neurologist at 27.
I was completely fed up and decided to rebuild at 28.

Like I said, I was a temple in ruins, with numerous bodily systems malfunctioning. But I have since studied the plan of the Architect and Creator, and I have begun to rebuild. While I am an on-going work in progress, I can happily report that I am no longer overweight (I lost every, single, dang, stubborn pound). I do not take any prescription medications. I no longer have reoccurring anxiety attacks or any symptoms of depression. I do not have any indications of my former heart issues. My blood pressure, cholesterol, and glucose are fantastic. I do not have any regular numbness, pain, or lightheadedness. And, given the fact that my focus used to be so bad I could not read a single page in a book, I would say that is better now too... considering this is the sixth book I've written in two years.

I relay all of this because I will suggest doing many hard things in this book. (Food prepping, counting macros, reading labels, giving up sugar! Blah, I know!) But please don't think I don't understand just how hard it is. Please know that I am writing from a "been there, done that" kind of place. Know that I'm writing more from my heart than my head. And remember, I'm a health _coach_ which means, I'm going to _coach_ you here in these pages. I'm going to ask you to dig deep, to work hard, to get back on the saddle when you fall (and you _will_ fall). I'm going to ask you to keep going and never to give up.

The fact that you picked up this book tells me somewhere in your heart you know something needs to change regarding your health... and I take that very seriously.

So, I will push you in these pages. As your coach, my expectations are high because my hope for you is high.

A Regenerating Machine

To be clear, in this book I am not claiming that any of these products or strategies or foods can cure, treat, prevent, or heal any disease or illness. But I do believe that God designed the body with its incredible ability to do this in various cases, given the right tools, materials, and environment.

You see, the body is in a constant state of regeneration. It is by its very nature a self-healing type of machine. This is illustrated in the fact that when you cut your finger, it typically doesn't remain an open wound forever. It scabs, and it heals. The same is true of a broken bone. In most cases, it doesn't remain broken forever, it heals. Now, I do realize there _are_ instances where "permanent damage" occurs, but that's not what I'm talking about here.

You see, there are trillions of cells in the human body. Each type of cell has its own "life span," so to speak. This life span differs depending on what type of cell it is. White blood cells, for example, can live for more than a year, but red blood cells can live for only about four months or so. Skin cells can live for approximately two or three weeks, but intestinal cells live for only a few days. In fact, it is said that the body replaces all the cells in the small intestine about every five days. That equals almost 17 billion new cells, six times a month!

Despite this, some of you are still despairing because of your discouraging genes. You look at your family history and want to throw in the towel. "What's the use?" you think. "I'm doomed." But even our genes do not fate us to disease in most cases. It's all about how genes express themselves, how they act in the body. And, friend, your diet has a very powerful ability to "turn off" genes that lead to disease and "turn on" genes that promote better health.

Like I said, the body was designed to be a regenerating machine. It was created by the God of _Life_, the Creator of all that is "good." This should give us even *more* hope. I'm guessing, if you started reading this book, you're looking for this hope, and looking for a change. Maybe you are looking to lose weight, have more energy, better mood, or easier digestion. Maybe you're looking for better lab results at your next annual wellness visit, or better skin, hair, and nails. Maybe you're looking to _stay_ healthy and not be a victim of age-related declining health.

Or maybe, just maybe, you feel like a steam engine coasting downhill. Maybe you're worried that, if something doesn't change, you won't live to see your kids get married or your grandkids grow up. Maybe you are at your wit's end because you have already tried so many other diets and strategies, without any success whatsoever. Maybe that has made you skeptical about reading this book (so you're now reading with a hint of cynicism and maybe even some eye-rolling).

If this is you, let me be the first to say: it's ok. I did the same thing once upon a time. But I'm confident *Rebuilding Your Temple* is unlike any other book you've picked up. And that, my friend, is a very good thing.

So, without further delay... let's start rebuilding, shall we?

References:

(1) https://www.cdc.gov/obesity/data/adult.html
(2) http://www.acc.org/latest-in-cardiology/ten-points-to-remember/2017/02/09/14/58/heart-disease-and-stroke-statistics-2017
(3) https://www.cancer.gov/about-cancer/understanding/statistics
(4) https://www.aarda.org/knowledge-base/many-americans-autoimmune-disease/
(5) https://www.cdc.gov/media/releases/2017/p0718-diabetes-report.html
(6) https://newsnetwork.mayoclinic.org/discussion/nearly-7-in-10-americans-take-prescription-drugs-mayo-clinic-olmsted-medical-center-find/

Phase 1:

Rebuilding the Fueling System

Materials Used in Phase 1: Quality fats and low-glycemic, complex carbohydrates

Tools to Consider for Phase 1: Plexus Slim, Plexus Slim Hunger Control, Plexus Block, Plexus Balance, and Plexus Active

Chapter 1: Consider Fat As Fuel

Disclaimer: These statements have not been evaluated by the Food and Drug Administration. None of the information in this book is intended to diagnose, treat, cure, or prevent any disease. All information contained in this chapter and this book is for educational purposes only and are not intended to replace the advice of a medical doctor. Stacy Malesiewski is not a doctor and does not give medical advice, prescribe medication, or diagnose illness. Stacy is a certified health coach, journalist, and an independent Plexus ambassador. These are her personal beliefs and are not the beliefs of Plexus Worldwide, Gray Matter Media, Inc., or any other named professionals in this book. If you have a medical condition or health concern, it is advised that you see your physician immediately. It is also recommended that you consult your doctor before implementing any new health strategy or taking any new supplements. Results may vary.

During the first phase of this renovation, we look at how to rebuild the temple's fueling system. The first step in doing that is to determine the *type* of fuel you want to use. A typical house usually has a furnace that handles the fuel—be it gas, electric, or propane. If it's a natural gas furnace, a pilot light ignites burners inside a combustion chamber, which makes heat. The heat enters a heat exchanger, where the heat transfers to the air via blowers and duct work.

But, what about the temple of the body? Do we have a "furnace" inside of us that can produce and distribute energy? Yes, we do. It's called the mitochondria, often referred to as the "powerhouse of the cell," and rightly so.

Like a furnace, mitochondria take oxygen from the air we breathe, as well as either glucose (from carbohydrates) or ketones (from fat), and they produce energy for our body, called adenosine triphosphate (or ATP as I'll refer to it from here on out). This is a super simplified analogy of a very complex process, but I think you get my drift. And while a house typically only has one furnace, the temple of the human body has many, MANY mitochondria in *each cell*!

Some cells have between 80 and 2,000 mitochondria, and other cells have hundreds of thousands of mitochondria. Your heart has more than 5,000 mitochondria per cell! So, these little "temple furnaces" are pumping out a lot of energy! Or at least, they should be. Some estimate the mitochondria can produce 110 pounds of ATP every day. Biochemist, Nick Lane, says they pump about 10,000 times more energy (gram for gram) than the sun every SECOND!! (1)

Clearly, then, if this is how we get our energy, it's important to provide these "temple furnaces" with a fuel they can use efficiently. Therefore, like a builder of a house, we first have to determine which type of primary fuel we want to use: either carbohydrates or fat. Before you make that decision, though, let's talk about the differences in detail so that you're well informed when you discuss this with your doctor.

First, let's start with ketones.

Let's look at the furnace of a house again. Newer model furnaces can run at high-efficiency levels, sometimes up to 98%. This basically means they turn 98% of the fuel they consume into heat. Compare that to an old coal or wood furnace from back in the day. Those weren't nearly as efficient—or clean. Some old furnaces had an efficiency rate of only 60%, and they produced really dirty soot as well.

This is like the temple furnace—the mitochondria. As I told you, the mitochondria can use either glucose or ketones for energy. But these fuels are not used in the same way. Mitochondria handle glucose like an old coal or wood furnace whereas they handle ketones like a high-efficiency natural gas furnace.

Let me explain.

First, fat (fatty acids) can get directly into the mitochondria intact, but carbs need to be broken down _outside_ the mitochondria before they can be transported inside. So, that makes fatty acids a more readily usable fuel. Second, you often get more energy per molecule of fat than you do per molecule of sugar, which is what carbs are essentially broken down to. In fact, 1g of stored fatty acids generates about six times as much ATP energy as does 1g of stored glucose. (2) So, not only is it more readily available, but it's also a more powerful fuel. If that wasn't enough, using fat as fuel actually creates additional mitochondria in the brain (3)—and more furnaces mean more brain power.

Third, all temple furnaces produce a residue or soot (just like a home furnace), regardless of the fuel that is used. As mitochondria make ATP energy, they produce what are called free radicals which can damage the cell, causing it to disintegrate. You can't prevent this from happening as it's a normal part of the process. It's just how it works. But, burning glucose is like using an old coal or wood furnace because it creates a lot more of these free radicals.

Plain and simple, glucose is a somewhat "dirty" fuel for the temple. This is especially true if you are eating the wrong kinds of carbs, which we will discuss in the next chapter. Burning fat, on the other hand, is often called a cleaner fuel because it can _inhibit_ the production of free radicals (the soot). In fact, it's estimated that burning ketones can lower mitochondria exposure to free radical damage by as much as 40%! (4)

While most people operate primarily on glucose fuel (carbohydrates), there is a growing number of people that are "switching fuels," so to speak. They are beginning to restrict carbohydrate intake and increase fat consumption. This is called a keto or ketogenic diet, sometimes referred to as a "low carb" diet or even a "low carb/high-fat diet."

When the temple makes this transition and begins to use fat/ketones as its primary fuel source (instead of carbs/glucose), it is called being in a state of ketosis. Once in ketosis, ketones are produced by the liver from fat and, as I said, are then used for energy.

But food is not the _only_ way this is accomplished. The body can also use _stored_ fat too—meaning, it can use the fat in your hips, belly, and buttocks as fuel for the body as well. It's taking belly fat and using it as brain power for that work deadline or using it for energy for your gym workout. In ketosis, you literally become a fat-burning machine. So, this can be enormously beneficial for those who are obese or trying to lose a significant amount of weight.

Other Reasons Why You Might Want to Switch Fuels

When your body uses glucose for energy, it's important to understand that glucose can't go directly into your cells like ketones can. It's not usable by itself. It needs insulin. Insulin is like the "key" that unlocks the door of the cell so that the glucose can get in to be used for energy.

Essentially, when you eat carbohydrates, those carbs turn into glucose. Your blood glucose (blood sugar) level then rises, and this tells your pancreas to release insulin. It is _insulin_, then, that attaches to the glucose and "unlocks" the cells to receive the glucose from the blood. So, in other words, without insulin, you simply cannot use glucose as fuel. And if you can't use glucose as fuel, you will not have energy, even while eating carbohydrates.

If we're talking furnaces again, I guess you could say insulin is like the pilot light on a furnace. The pilot light provides the flame needed to light the gas and make heat. It "turns on" the furnace, so to speak. If there's no pilot light, the natural gas isn't really "usable." Likewise, if there's no insulin, the glucose isn't usable. It just accumulates and circulates in the bloodstream.

Now, if you eat more carbs or sugar than you need for energy at that moment, insulin will also help store the leftover glucose in your liver, to be used later when you need it. Glucose in the liver can also be turned into glycogen and stored in muscles for later use too. But, the thing is, the liver and muscles have a _limited_ capacity. They can only store so much of it. So, any glucose that exceeds the energy needs or storage capacity is then converted to and stored as _fat_! And, unfortunately, the body has NO LIMIT in fat storage. This is how eating too many carbs can lead to weight gain.

For many people, this is what originally damaged their temple fueling system — consuming too much dirty fuel. How exactly does this cause damage? Well, when you overindulge in sugar and processed carbohydrates day in and day out for many years, it can cause blood sugar imbalances.

Eating too many carbs can spike your blood sugar levels too high. And the pancreas isn't good under pressure. So, when it gets the red flag that there's too much sugar in the bloodstream, it often works too hard, sending out too much insulin (to start unlocking cells and moving to storage). Unfortunately, this can end up lowering the blood sugar level too low. Then when it's too low, the body thinks that you're starving, so it sends out the signal to eat again, to raise the glucose level in the blood. And often, that means _overeat_ because the low blood sugar level makes you feel famished.

Overeating then spikes blood sugar levels too high again, the pancreas sends too much insulin, and the vicious cycle continues on and on. Because insulin is one of the most powerful hormones in the body, this erratic insulin production can lead to other hormone imbalances, which I will talk about later in this book.

It can also cause what's known as Insulin Resistance. Insulin resistance is when cells start resisting or ignoring insulin. Insulin becomes like "the boy who cried wolf," and cells no longer respond to the signals it sends to "open up." So, the pancreas sends even more and more insulin, like some biological attempt to "yell louder" at the cells.

Over time, though, the insulin-producing cells in the pancreas get tired and worn out. They become less and less able to meet these insulin demands of the body, brought on by the high carb diet. The result: glucose stays in the bloodstream, and you end up with high blood sugar all the time—aka, type 2 diabetes. And that's not all it can lead to. Insulin resistance also plays a role in obesity, hypertension, dyslipidemia, polycystic ovarian syndrome (PCOS), and cardiovascular disease.

What's more, high sugar/carb intake can make brain cells insulin resistant, too, which can cause those cells to die, as well. It's not surprising, then, that Alzheimer's disease has been dubbed, "Type 3 Diabetes" in recent years. Abnormal glucose levels can also cause seizures. They result in altered glucose metabolism, as well as a reduction of ATP. This is why a no-sugar ketogenic diet is often used as a therapy for Epilepsy.

Contrary to the belief of some, the ketogenic diet is not just a fad or some unfounded craze. Because of ground-breaking research, it is gaining the attention and approval of some of the most prominent medical experts—and not just as it relates to Epilepsy. Many well-known professionals are becoming strong, outspoken proponents of the ketogenic diet for other health conditions too. A few of these doctors (my favorites) include:

- Dr. Joseph Mercola DO—Osteopathic physician and New York Times best-selling author (www.mercola.com)
- Dr. Anna Cabeca—a triple board-certified Ob-Gyn and women's health expert, Amazon #1 best-selling author (www.drannacabeca.com)
- Dr. David Jockers DNM, DC, MS—Doctor of natural medicine, functional nutritionist and corrective care chiropractor (www.drjockers.com)
- Dr. Josh Axe, DC, DNM, CNS—Doctor of chiropractic, certified doctor of natural medicine and clinical nutritionist (www.draxe.com)
- Dr. Mark Hyman, MD—a practicing family physician, a ten-time #1 New York Times bestselling author, Director the Cleveland Clinic Center for Functional Medicine, and founder and medical director of The UltraWellness Center (www.drhyman.com)
- Dr. Tom O'Bryan, DC, CCN, DACBN—an internationally recognized speaker, international docuseries host, writer and expert on chronic disease and metabolic disorders, with teaching faculty positions at the Institute for Functional Medicine and the National University of Health Sciences, and more than 30 years of experience as a functional medicine practitioner and educator (www.thedr.com)
- Dr. Amy Myers MD—a renowned leader in functional medicine specializing in women's health issues (particularly gut health, thyroid dysfunction, and autoimmunity), and two-time New York Times bestselling author (www.amymyersmd.com)
- Dr. David Perlmutter, MD, FACN—Board-Certified Neurologist and four-time New York Times bestselling author, and the recipient of the Linus Pauling Award (among others) for his innovative approaches to neurological disorders (www.drperlmutter.com)
- Dr. Eric Berg, DC—a chiropractor and author whose patients have included senior officials in the U.S. government and the Justice Department, ambassadors, among others. He is on the advisory panel for the Health Science Institute and has worked as a past part-time adjunct professor at Howard University. (www.drberg.com)
- Jill C. Carnahan, MD, ABIHM, IFMCP—Board certified in both Family Medicine and Integrative Holistic Medicine, a functional medicine consultant, speaker, writer, and media personality (www.jillcarnahan.com)

I strongly encourage you to explore the wealth of information that these aforementioned doctors have made available to the public. These and many other professionals are speaking out about the benefits of a ketogenic diet for a host of chronic health conditions. Some of these include:

- obesity
- insulin resistance
- diabetes
- hypertension and heart disease
- regular seizures
- conditions like dementia, Alzheimer's or Parkinson's
- lack of focus and mental clarity
- yeast overgrowth
- cancer (especially of the brain, nervous system and blood))
- chronic pain

If you have the above conditions and are interested in adopting the ketogenic diet, you must speak with your doctor about this information. **This is especially true if you have diabetes, as your doctor may need to adjust your insulin dose if you plan to remove carbohydrates from your diet.**

That being said, even though ketosis can be extremely beneficial for many people, there are some instances when it might _not_ be a good idea. Even the doctors mentioned above all agree that it is not for everyone. No diet is. Therefore, if you fall into any of the below categories, it is especially important to discuss the keto risks with your doctor:

- Pregnant or breastfeeding women: women who are expecting a child or who have just given birth should not try a strict ketogenic diet. However, some pregnant/breastfeeding women do well on a modified, lower carb eating plan of fewer than 100 grams (gr) of carbohydrates per day. But this absolutely must be approved by an obstetrician beforehand.
- Children or teenagers: most children and teens should not try a ketogenic diet except in cases of cancer, epilepsy, obesity, or insulin resistance. In those cases, it can be beneficial, but it is imperative first to discuss it with a pediatrician.
- Those with unmanaged Adrenal Fatigue: while a ketogenic diet has proven very beneficial for various stress-related issues, those who suffer from adrenal fatigue that is not well managed may need to ease into ketosis, or cycle in and out of it, depending on how extreme symptoms are. They also may need to do a modified keto plan, eating slightly more carbs, at least at the beginning.
- Genetic mutations, especially regarding the ApoE gene: The ApoE gene gives the body directions on how to make a special protein that combines with

fats to form lipoproteins (which carry cholesterol through the bloodstream). Put simply; this gene determines how your body metabolizes cholesterol. People with an ApoE variant (specifically ApoE4) can experience elevated cholesterol while eating a high *saturated* fat diet. However, that does not necessarily mean keto is out of the question because a high monounsaturated fat diet can have the opposite effect. If you are concerned that you have this gene variation, ask your doctor about genetic testing. You can also order your own genetic testing online through companies such as 23andMe®. However, understanding your genetics is complex, so if you take this route, you should also consider genetic counseling.

- Those with a low functioning thyroid: depending on the root cause of the thyroid disorder, severe carb restriction (like a ketogenic diet) can potentially make thyroid function worse (especially if it is related to adrenal fatigue.) In this case, some find a moderately low carb/high-protein diet to be more beneficial than a severely low carb diet. I will talk about this in the next chapter also. Those with an overactive thyroid, however, may benefit from a ketogenic diet as research has shown high-fat consumption lowers the thyroid hormone Triiodothyronine (T3). (5)

- Those with liver issues: The liver is the main organ involved in metabolizing fat for energy, so if your liver is impaired in any way, it is important to discuss this with your doctor before implementing a ketogenic diet. Your practitioner may advise you to take some form of liver support supplement, such as the one offered by Dr. Myers on her website. (https://store.amymyersmd.com)

- Those with hypertension: while the ketogenic diet has been proven to be very anti-inflammatory and assist with dramatic weight loss (both of which can help hypertension), some people have a genetic makeup that causes a higher sodium intake. This could be problematic if the high fat "keto" foods you are eating are high in sodium as this can *increase* blood pressure. For this reason, it is crucial to stay in close contact with your doctor (perhaps even discussing potassium supplementation). It is also important to choose healthy *anti-inflammatory* fats, which I will discuss in Phase 2. Lastly, if you smoke, be aware that nicotine can raise blood pressure 15-20 units. It may not be that "keto isn't right" for you, it may be simply that you need to quit nicotine.

- Those who have had their gallbladder removed: The job of the gallbladder is to store and concentrate bile, made from the liver. Bile is a liquid that works with lipase enzymes from the pancreas to break down and dissolve fat in the digestive system. So, as you can imagine, bile is very important on a ketogenic diet when 75-80% of calories come from fat. Without a gallbladder, there is no storage or concentration of bile, just a slower flow of bile from the liver where it is made. This means there is a possibility that without a gallbladder, there could be a shortage of bile or bile that is not concentrated enough to do its job. If you do not have a gallbladder but are still interested in the ketogenic diet, it is important to talk to your doctor about a bile salts supplement, such as those from Dr. Berg or Dr. Mercola.

- Those who already have elevated cholesterol: This is one of the main concerns that people have when they hear that keto is a "high-fat diet," especially those who already struggle with cholesterol issues. If the cholesterol problems are genetic (from an ApoE variant like I mentioned above) this is a valid concern. However, if it is not related to genes, it's important to consider all factors. There is much more to high cholesterol than meets the eye. In fact, a *low*-fat diet can sometimes be more dangerous than nutritional ketosis, which I will discuss in later chapters. In the meantime, if you have elevated cholesterol or fear that you might develop it if you adopt a ketogenic diet, talk to your doctor beforehand. I also ***highly recommend*** reading an article called "High Cholesterol on a Ketogenic Diet" by Dr. Jockers. It is one of the most simplified and well-written pieces I've come across on the subject and can be found at this address: https://drjockers.com/high-cholesterol-ketogenic-diet/

What You Can and Cannot Eat on a Ketogenic Diet

Perhaps by now, you are intrigued about the ketogenic diet, but you are not sure what you can eat if you adopt this plan. We will talk more about this (in great detail) in later chapters but below is a basic list of "Dos and Don'ts." This list will evolve a great deal, though, as we go through different phases, so please don't stop reading here.

What You Can Eat on a Ketogenic Diet	What You Cannot Eat on a Ketogenic Diet
MCT oil	
Olive oil	Cow Milk
Eggs	Rice Milk
Butter	Flavored milk
Ghee	Coffee creamer
Coconut oil	Cottage cheese
Coconut (unsweetened)	Yogurt of any kind
Unsweetened almond milk	American cheese
Coconut milk	Bottled salad dressings
Most cheese	Wheat flour or baking mix

Full fat sour cream	Gluten-free flour or baking mix
Full fat cream cheese	Any wheat product
Whipping cream	Bread
Salmon	Pasta
Beef	Potatoes
Tuna	Sweet potatoes
Fish	Quinoa
Chicken	Beans or lentils
Plain pork	Rice of any kind
Natural sugar-free bacon	Oatmeal or granola
Shrimp	Grits
Vinegar (red wine, white, apple cider)	Boxed cereal
Mayonnaise	Tomatoes
Mustard	Marinara sauce
Braggs amino acids	Ketchup
Worcestershire sauce	Barbeque sauce
Red Hot	Crackers
Lemons	Chips or pretzels
Celery	Health bars
Onions	Fruits
Mushrooms	Juice
Lettuce of any kind	Sugar of any kind
Cucumbers	Artificial Sweeteners
Cauliflower	Corn Syrup
Yellow squash	Fructose
Zucchini	Smoked meats
Broccoli	Salsa
Coffee	Jar cheese sauce
Stevia (liquid is best)	Hummus
Monk fruit	Wraps
Xylitol	Tortillas
Erythritol	Honey
Almond flour	Syrup of any kind
Coconut flour	Agave
Pasta zero	Soda (even sugar-free kind)
Pork rinds	Alcohol
Chia seeds	Low-calorie drinks (except Plexus
Dill pickles	Slim)
Avocado	
Cabbage	

The following is a list of foods that are not necessarily *restricted* on the ketogenic diet but require you use caution because they could contain hidden sugars, chemicals, or carbs. For this reason, it is important to READ LABELS carefully and only eat these foods in moderation.

- Deli meats (many have sugar and chemicals)
- Bratwurst or sausage links (most have sugar and harmful chemicals)
- Peanut Butter (has some carbs/sugar)
- Nut butter (some carbs)
- Nuts (some have carbs, though pecans are lower)
- Seeds (while seeds are a favorite part of my keto diet, some types have carbs, others do not)
- Bell Peppers (contains sugar)
- Carrots (carbs and sugar)
- Beef jerky (hidden sugars)
- Spaghetti squash (carbs)
- Protein Powders (Plexus P96 is ok)

Hold Up! What About Alcohol?

Some of you may have seen alcohol listed in the "No-No" column and are now concerned. Maybe you're asking, "Can't I still drink alcohol and go keto?" The answer is yes... and no. It is a slippery slope.

Here's the thing: when you drink alcohol, your body is getting the signal that there is something toxic present. The liver uses all the body's resources to process the toxin as quickly as possible, which takes away from other processes, like fat oxidation (aka ketone production). Basically, your body is going to burn the alcohol before it burns anything else. So, regardless of what kind of alcohol you drink, alcohol can interfere with the keto diet (any diet, really). It might not totally prevent it from working, but it definitely will make it more difficult.

That being said, there are certain types of alcohol that "might" be "ok," and then there are certain types of alcohol that just plain won't work at all. So, let's go over it.

Let's start with beer. Barley is the main ingredient in beer (a grain with carbs). It is broken down to maltose (which is sugar), which the yeast acts on. So, no matter which way you slice it, beer by its very nature is anti-keto. Even low carb beer might kick you out of ketosis. So, it may be beneficial to stay away from those as well.

Wine is a little different. It's made from grapes—which are carbs and sugar, yes—but the yeast consumes most of the sugar in the grapes and converts it to ethanol and carbon dioxide, so there's not as much sugar left, like say, a grape juice or something. But there still is sugar present. Sweet wines obviously have quite a bit more sugar left. But even dry wines have "some" sugar which could affect ketosis for some people. Some estimate there is almost 1 gram of carbs per ounce of dry wine.

Even still, it probably isn't a good idea to drink a sweet wine while trying to switch fuels and get into ketosis, but it might not even be a good idea to try a dry wine the first couple weeks... at least before you are fully "keto-adapted" and your body gets used to your new diet. You don't want sugar present when you're trying to "train" your body to use a different fuel source.

Pure spirits like whiskey and vodka contain zero carbs. But again, your body is going to burn the alcohol first, which can slow ketosis. Also, you need to consider mixers. Traditional soda is not something I ever advocate. (We will talk about the reasons later.) Even "diet" versions of most soda are full of ingredients that wreak havoc on the body.

So, what _can_ you drink in terms of mixers? You could try club soda, or maybe make your own soda using a carbonation machine and flavored liquid stevia drops. (Sweet Leaf® brand even makes a root beer flavor.) You can also brew your own homemade iced tea with flavored tea bags. Or you could sweeten regular tea with flavored stevia drops.

You might also consider products like La Croix® (carbonated water and natural fruit oils with no carbs and no sugar) and Zevia® (a soda made with Stevia and erythritol that has only four carbs and no sugar). The body can't break down/metabolize erythritol, so this is a keto-safe option.

Basically, alcohol is somewhat of a gray area in terms of ketosis. Some people can handle a glass or two of dry wine; some people can't. Some people can have pure spirits with a low-calorie mixer; some people don't feel good doing so. If you want to play it safe, I would avoid alcohol at the beginning—especially if you have a candida yeast overgrowth.

I will talk a lot more about candida in later chapters. But for now, in terms of alcohol, it's important to know that candida is a harmful yeast that can use ethanol (alcohol) as an energy source. So, when you drink alcohol, it is like giving candida an IV of the very thing it lives on. This then can make a yeast infection or overgrowth worse.

Second, your liver is a key player in fighting candida. It is responsible for getting rid of the 70 different toxins and byproducts associated with candida (like acetaldehyde, uric acid, and ammonia, among other things). But, drinking alcohol puts extra stress on the liver. So, drinking while trying to fight candida can overwork your liver, which could result in toxin buildup and some unwanted detox symptoms.

It's also important to note that candida and alcohol often go hand in hand. As I said, when you eat sugar/carbs, candida can convert it into alcohol/ethanol for energy. If you consume alcohol on top of this, it can cause strong cravings for _more_ alcohol, which can make it hard to stop drinking after just one glass. This is why it is very common for alcoholics also to have a candida overgrowth... though it's the classic questions of, "which came first the chicken or the egg?"

My point is: even if you do find a type of alcohol that is low carb and low sugar, it should be consumed in moderation (or not at all) because of the negative impact it has on overall health. Also, be forewarned: you may be a "cheap date" drinking while in ketosis. It is not uncommon for you to feel a "buzz" much earlier than you normally would using glucose as fuel.

It may be best to avoid alcohol at least until you are keto-adapted or until the candida is cleared up. But, if you can't do this—if you have special occasions where it just can't be avoided—make sure you choose an option with the lowest sugar possible.

When You're on the Go or Traveling

Some of you may be very interested in switching fuels but are worried about whether you can keep up with this kind of diet when you're on the go or traveling. This is a very legitimate concern. It can be difficult to eat keto on the road, or at a restaurant with friends. But it is not impossible. Here are some tips that can help.

1.) Salads: Most restaurants offer a salad or two that are keto-friendly. A cobb salad, for example, is an excellent choice because of the meats, cheeses, and eggs, even guacamole! If a salad comes with breaded chicken, ask for it grilled instead. Also, many sub shops will make their subs into salads if you ask. Just ask for oil and vinegar for the dressing.

2.) Plain Food: Order a side of steamed "seasonal" vegetables (usually broccoli and cauliflower etc.) and a meat option (steak, chicken, salmon). Tell your waiter you have "dietary restrictions" and ask them to cook your food with just butter and seasons, no sauces.

3.) All Day Breakfast: Find a restaurant that serves all-day breakfast and order bacon and eggs or an omelet loaded with bacon, cheese, etc.

4.) Wings: Choose a restaurant that sells chicken wings. You can order parmesan, dry ranch, or butter and garlic wings with celery sticks and sour cream, as these are keto-friendly. Most other wing sauces such as barbecue sauce have a lot of sugar, though so I do not recommend those.

5.) Go Bun-less: You can order a burger (or grilled chicken sandwich) without the bun! Have them load it up with lettuce, cheese, onions, bacon, mushrooms, etc. Order a side salad or seasonal veggies with it and grab a fork!

6.) Mexican: Order fajitas or tacos without the wraps/shells. Just ask for extra lettuce and put the "goodies" over the lettuce like a salad. Add sour cream and guacamole for a nice dressing. Some restaurants offer fajita bowls too. Just skip the rice and beans and add extra avocado.

7.) Nuggets: Grilled (unbreaded) chicken tenders or nuggets are also a safe keto option if you are in a pinch. I'm not a fan of fast food (AT ALL), but I understand there are times when you're limited in offerings, especially when it comes to traveling.

8.) Chinese: You also might consider ordering a stir fry at a Chinese buffet. Look for one that has a make-your-own grill. Just load up your veggies and meats and ask the chef to grill it in just butter and garlic—no sauces, as they typically contain a lot of sugar and unhealthy ingredients too.

The Downfalls of Transitioning

Maybe you're getting excited about the possibility of what a ketogenic lifestyle can do for you; maybe you want to get started right away. That's awesome. But hang on a minute. We need to talk about transitioning.

Before your body can begin using ketones as its primary fuel, it first must use up all the available and _stored_ glucose. Remember how I told you that insulin not only unlocks cells to receive glucose but also transports glucose to storage? Well, that means that even if you stop eating carbs, you will still be using glucose fuel for a little while because you'll be using what is stored. And this could be substantial. Dr. Hyman estimates that we have "about 2,500 calories of carbohydrate (in the form of glycogen) stored in our muscles." (To find out more, watch his podcast The Doctor's Farmacy at drhyman.com/blog/2018/09/05/podcast-ep17/)

Once you use up stored glucose, your body will eventually enter a state of ketosis and begin to use ketones for fuel, if they are readily available. However, as the carbohydrate fuel depletes to lower and lower levels, you could start to experience some negative side effects, commonly referred to as the keto flu. The most common sign is fatigue because you're "running on empty" so to speak.

You can also experience brain fog, headache, irritability, sugar cravings, and an upset stomach. This is common, and it's a good sign! It means you've almost switched fuels. But, yes, it can be uncomfortable and inconvenient. So, you need to plan accordingly.

For most people, this lasts only about a half of a day (maybe an entire day, or even a day and a half, depending on the person*). But then, boom! When you fully switch over into ketosis, you often get a burst of energy using your new high-efficiency fuel.

But, again, you must plan for that uncomfortable "in-between" phase. You might not want to have brain fog or fatigue on a day when you have a big work meeting, a college exam, or if you need to drive 10 hours. So, for some people, it might be best to stop eating carbs on Friday so that you transition over the weekend and start fresh at work on Monday. Or maybe you have a busy weekend with a lot going on, and it would be easier for you to start transitioning on a Wednesday so that you are back to feeling good before Friday. Regardless, you need to look at your calendar and plan when would be best for you to start the keto diet. Do not just jump into this without consulting your doctor or planning appropriately.

If you do experience the Keto-Flu, though, here are some common strategies that seem to help many people:

1. First, don't give up! Remember it's short-lived, and it's a good sign!!!
2. Replenish electrolytes by drinking more water, and eat more healthy fats
3. Try 8/16 intermittent fasting, as it can help speed up ketosis. This means eating for only 8 hours (say from 7 AM to 3 PM or 10 AM to 6 PM) then fasting for 16 hours until the next morning. We will talk much more about this in future chapters.
4. Exercise! Using up stored glucose during exercise will help you get into ketosis faster.

Some people who are severely carb addicted or have other preexisting health issues could potentially experience the Keto-Flu for several days, even a week. Please stay in touch with your doctor if is you!

How Will I know?

As I've already mentioned, there are many benefits to a ketogenic diet. But most of the benefits are a result of being in a state of ketosis, not just eating more fat.

There's a big difference. While eating healthy fats is certainly beneficial, it is _not_ the same as _using fat as fuel_. Some people make the mistake of dramatically increasing fat consumption, but they don't limit carbs so they never "switch fuels." They don't become a fat-burning machine because they remain a glucose burning machine. And if you're not burning all the extra fat you're consuming; you could be storing it. So, it's very important to make sure that you are in a nutritional state of ketosis.

But how can you "really" know if you are in a state of ketosis or not? First, measure ketones. You see, there are three types of ketones in the body: Acetoacetate, β-Hydroxybutyrate (BHB), and Acetone. Each of these is measured by a different means, so you don't have to guess.

Acetone is produced quickly, sometimes as soon as you start to transition. It's a highly volatile ketone body that can be exhaled, so it is most often measured on your breath with a ketone meter breathalyzer. You can purchase one of these for as low as $20, or up to $280, depending on the device. But sometimes, you don't even need a breathalyzer. Sometimes you can just "taste" the transition into ketosis. It's often described as a fruity taste in your mouth. Others may even comment your breath smells metallic. This is often referred to as "keto breath." Both are indicators that acetone ketones are present, which is a good sign that you are transitioning into ketosis.

If you are concerned about keto breath, though, do not just go out and buy a regular pack of gum or breath mints. There is often sugar in these, and so many brands can inhibit ketosis. Below is a list of other keto-friendly options:

> 1.) Add a drop of natural, therapeutic grade peppermint, spearmint or cinnamon essential oils to your glass of water
>
> 2.) Make a homemade breath spray by mixing 2-5 drops of essential oils with purified water and a dash of sea salt in a 4 oz spray bottle.
>
> 3.) Make your own "fat mints" by mixing melted or softened coconut oil with essential oils and granulated stevia. Spoon onto wax paper or into molds and refrigerate until hardened.

Another way to measure ketones is to test your urine. This can be done by purchasing a 30 or 60-day pack of ketone urine strips at your local drug store or online at various shopping sites like Amazon.com. They cost approximately $10-$15 and are easy to use (you just pee on a stick).

But they do have some pitfalls.

Urine strips only measure _excess_ acetoacetate ketone bodies—meaning the ones that are leftover, that are not used by the body and therefore excreted through urine. Urine ketone strips are very helpful at the beginning of the ketogenic diet because they can tell you precisely whether or not you're in a state of ketosis. But, once you become fat-adapted, and you begin to use fat more efficiently (say after four weeks or so), you may not have many acetoacetate ketones "leftover." You may be using everything you're making. So, the strips may not detect ketones anymore, even though you _are_ still in a state of ketosis.

Dehydration can also negatively affect urine results, as can testing right after exercise or eating. Also, it's not uncommon to get a batch of faulty strips. I've had many clients suffer great disappointment at the beginning of their transition— hoping and praying they were in nutritional ketosis, but nothing showed up in the urine. Sometimes if the strips get wet, heated, or damaged during shipping, they might not work anymore. So, if you aren't seeing results after a week, the first thing I usually do is buy new strips and re-test.

The third (and most accurate) way to test for ketones, is to test your blood for beta-hydroxybutyrate using a blood ketone meter. While acetone indicates early signs of ketosis and acetoacetate indicates leftovers, BHB indicates useable fuel. It's similar to a gas gauge in your car, measuring precisely what you've got to work with. Blood ketone meters are more expensive than breathalyzers and urine test strips, though. The meter itself can cost $50-$100, but the test strips can cost $5 apiece or more.

Regardless, I highly recommend testing in some way. You don't want to assume you're in ketosis when you're not. It's important to know. I personally used the urine strips at the beginning of my transition, and I never really needed to use other testing methods. I have been in nutritional ketosis for so long now that I know immediately when I switch back to using glucose, just by the way I feel.

Ketone Supplements

One of the questions health professionals hear a lot is, "Can't I just take ketones?" Obviously, I am a big fan of nutritional ketosis (I love ketones!), or I wouldn't have dedicated the first chapter of this book to it. But I'm not as big a fan of _taking_ ketones, at least at the beginning. Allow me to explain.

First, ketone supplementation (which is EXOgenous) is NOT THE SAME THING as being in a state of _nutritional_ ketosis from your diet (which is ENDOgenous ketone production that takes place in the liver).

Now, don't get me wrong, supplementing with exogenous ketones can have some fantastic benefits for people who are already in nutritional ketosis and who need a quick brain boost or energy lift. Medical professionals agree that it can also be great for people with Parkinson's, Alzheimer's, Epilepsy, ALS, Huntington's, or other degenerative neurological conditions, or people who have cancer who are following a nutritional ketogenic diet already. It can also prove beneficial for endurance athletes who need a lot more fuel than their food can provide.

But it's risky to think that you can just supplement with ketones while still eating carbs and experience the same wonderful effects as being in a state of nutritional ketosis. Research on this is in its early (very infant) stages, and we need much more data to understand the long-term effects of combining high amounts of ketones with high or moderate amounts carbohydrates. So far, at the publication of this book, I have not found enough data available to show that it is as beneficial as some are claiming. But currently, based on what I have found, it seems ketones are best when they ASSIST nutritional ketosis, not REPLACE it.

Here's the reasoning:

Through diet-induced nutritional ketosis, the body not only burns fat; it also does some pretty amazing and health-promoting things. It produces antioxidants, like glutathione, which Dr. Hyman calls the "mother of all antioxidants." Glutathione not only helps get rid of free radicals, but it also helps the immune system fight infections and plays a critical role in detoxification.

Nutritional ketosis also activates a family of proteins called Sirtuins needed for energy metabolism, DNA repair, inflammation regulation, and immune response. During ketosis, the body removes damaged cells (a process called autophagy), and it reduces amyloid-beta (plaque) in the brain (which is linked with Alzheimer's Disease). These are just a few of the many things that happen during _nutritional_ ketosis, which don't necessarily happen when just merely supplementing with ketones.

Therefore, when considering ketone supplementation, it's important to remember that doing things the right way often produces the best results. There are no shortcuts to true health, friends. You can't continue to carb-load, take ketones, and hope it serves as a loophole to ketosis.

That being said, if you are diligently following a clean ketogenic lifestyle and want to supplement with ketones to assist your energy needs, that's a different story. In those cases, ketone supplementation has proven to provide many benefits, but as always, it is important to discuss this with your doctor first.

Cheating on Keto

Some of you may be wondering how strict you have to be if you choose to adopt the ketogenic diet. You may be wondering if you can "cheat" here and there with a high carb meal, and still benefit. Maybe you've even heard that some people follow what's called a "Cyclical Ketogenic Diet," which means you "eat keto" for approximately five days followed by a couple of days of eating higher amounts of carbohydrates, such as on the weekend. Or some people go longer. They maintain ketosis for 7-10 days, then they cheat.

Carb cycling can be very beneficial. This is especially true for women if carbs are coordinated with the menstrual cycle (even the week following menstruation) because estrogen and progesterone impact carb metabolism. It can also be very beneficial for those with a low functioning thyroid, as I mentioned earlier.

It can also help bodybuilders, and other athletes refill muscle glycogen stores after long periods of carb restriction. And while ketosis has been shown to *boost* the hypothalamic-pituitary-adrenal (HPA) axis (which we'll talk about in later chapters), *long-term* carb restriction can stress out the HPA axis causing fatigue. It can inhibit mucus production, causing dry eyes and nasal passages. Therefore, carb cycling can be very healthy.

However, it's important not to reintroduce too many carbs before you reach a state of ketosis, or before you are keto-adapted. Also, carb cycling doesn't mean eating a box of Lucky Charms or a bag of Doritos. No. Carb cycling means eating *healthy* carbs, which we'll talk about in the next chapter. Again, carb cycling is for those who have been following a ketogenic diet (with their doctor's permission) and who are keto-adapted.

Carb-cycling before your body has adapted to the new fuel may not be a good idea because of the following reasons:

1.) It Will Kick You Out of Ketosis.

Cheating on the keto diet more than likely will kick you out of a state of ketosis— and at the beginning, it might take you some time to get back into ketosis. So, you "lose days" essentially. You might think, *"oh, well, that's ok. As long as I get back into ketosis after that."* But here's the thing: it's not *just* about being in ketosis. It's about efficiency. It's about training your body to be fat-adapted, to "habitually" burn fat for fuel. Your body isn't going to be adapted or efficient at anything if you're roller-coasting between glucose and fat every couple of days.

The more fat-adapted you are, and the more efficiently you burn fat as fuel, the more weight you will lose and the more health benefits you will see. Plain and simple. And it's important to remember a lot is going on "behind the scenes" when you enter ketosis. Your body makes changes (like altering hormones and increasing enzyme production among many other things) to improve conditions for burning fat. Having cheat meals regularly can prevent your body from doing this, so you won't be gaining the full health benefits that come from ketosis.

2.) Cheat Meals Will Spike Your Blood Sugar.

The keto diet is great for stabilizing blood glucose, as I already mentioned. But eating cheat meals (with carbs) will cause blood sugar levels to rise. Depending on how many you eat, this can cause fat storage and increased free radical production. Two of the primary goals of this protocol are to DECREASE free radical production and burn fat, not store it. Another goal is to address insulin resistance, to help cells become more sensitive to the presence of insulin. Having regular cheat meals makes it more difficult to reach these goals.

3.) You Make It Harder on Your Taste Buds.

As you begin to eat more fat and fewer carbs, your taste buds also adapt to the ketogenic diet. After a while, real food—especially healthy fats—become what tastes best. When you interrupt this process with more carb-heavy cheat foods, it can be like resetting your taste buds again. Garbage in, garbage out. And yes, you might get back into ketosis more easily after cheating, but you also may have some serious cravings for a little while because your taste buds aren't keto-adapted yet.

4.) Cheating Risks Keto-Flu.

Remember, the more carbs you eat on your cheat meal, the more carbs you will store and then have to burn off before you can start burning fat again—that means the longer it will take you to get back into ketosis, and the more likely you are to experience keto flu symptoms again. The fewer carbs you eat on a cheat meal, the quicker (and easier) you will get back into ketosis. When you go from strict keto to cheat meals—and back and forth—you could experience on-going keto flu symptoms like fatigue, headaches, low energy, migraines, and bloating.

That being said, if you do have a weak moment, and you do end up cheating, do not beat yourself up about it. Get back on the horse and start again. Try not to have the attitude of, "Well, I'm already out of ketosis; I may as well binge." You're only prolonging ketosis again.

To prevent future on-going cheating, try to think about WHY you cheated last time. Was it stress eating in response to something that happened? Was it because you got too hungry or because you didn't have enough healthy fat options on hand? Whatever the reason, try to address that underlying reason so that it doesn't happen again.

If you are a female and you are craving carbs because of monthly hormone fluctuations, prepare for that. Make chocolate fat bombs if you are a chocolate lover or make zucchini chips if you have a salty tooth. In any case: prepare, prepare, prepare!

Replace Don't Erase

If you've been reading this chapter, wanting to try the ketogenic diet but are afraid because your cravings for carbs are strong, let me say two things: One, that may be an indicator that you actually DO need to switch fuels. Ketosis can be a very successful strategy for breaking carb addictions. Two, my philosophy is, "Replace. Don't erase." That means, don't go cold turkey and completely erase all your favorite (unhealthy) foods from your diet right off the bat. You'll likely fail. It is better to replace those unhealthy favorites with healthier versions or alternatives. Let's face it: food is enjoyable. And it should be.

The key is to think about what you crave and how often, and then come up with replacements. For example*:

- If you love fajita bowls with white rice, replace the white rice with minced cauliflower rice.
- If you love ice cream and milkshakes, replace it with a low-carb, no-sugar, homemade milkshakes. *
- If you love chocolate and candy, make your own sugar free chocolate fat bombs.
- If you love baked goods like muffins, bread, and pancakes, make your own using keto-friendly flours such as almond flour and coconut flour.
- If you love hot gooey pizza, make your own with a keto crust or purchase a frozen one.
- If you love all kinds of potato chips, try switching to pork rinds or making your own salted zucchini chips.

*See the Rebuilding Your Temple Workbook for sample recipes.

References:

(1) http://nick-lane.net/wp-content/uploads/2017/01/Power-Sex-Suicide---Part-2.-The-Vital-Force-Proton-Power-and-the-Origin-of-Life.pdf
(2) https://www.ncbi.nlm.nih.gov/books/NBK21624/
(3) https://www.ncbi.nlm.nih.gov/pubmed/16807920
(4) Dr. Joseph Mercola; *Fat for Fuel A Revolutionary Diet to Combat Cancer, Boost Brain Power, and Increase Your Energy;* 2017 Carlsbad, CA; Hay House, Inc.; page 9
(5) https://www.ncbi.nlm.nih.gov/pubmed/3900181

Chapter 2: Consider Glucose Balance

If you are unable to adopt a ketogenic diet because of personal reasons, a doctor's recommendation, or a health condition, and you need to stick with glucose as your primary fuel, that is perfectly ok. Don't fret. It's still possible to rebuild the temple fueling system and increase efficiency _without_ switching fuels. It's simply about maintaining glucose balance, which we will discuss at length in this chapter. Also, please do not skip this chapter if you have already decided to go keto. I encourage you to research BOTH fuels first and then make an informed decision with the health of your doctor.

What's more, this chapter will contain valuable information for those who decide to carb cycle after becoming fat-adapted on the ketogenic diet. It will also be helpful for those who decide to switch back to using glucose again after a certain amount of time in ketosis. This information on glucose balance is also very important if you are a parent or caretaker who must cook and meal plan for others.

Now, let's talk glucose. Glucose, as we mentioned, comes from carbohydrates. But _not_ all carbohydrates are created equal! The Architect of your temple designed the body to run on _specific_ carbohydrates—complex carbohydrates and simple carbohydrates. These are far different from refined carbohydrates. Like propane and natural gas, they might "seem" similar at first glance, but they are not. Allow me to explain.

You see, carbohydrates are made up of three components: fiber, starch, and sugar. Fiber and starch are complex carbs. They digest slowly over time, and so they supply a very _steady_ source of energy for the body. Complex carbs are found in foods like peas, beans, whole grains, and vegetables.

Sugar is a simple carb. Simple carbs are broken down very quickly by the body to be used for a more immediate source of energy. They are found naturally in foods like fruits, milk, and other dairy products. To recap: complex carbs are steady carbs; simple carbs are quick carbs. Both are healthy forms of carbohydrates used for different needs.

Then, there are refined or processed carbohydrates. These carbs are carbs you won't find in nature. They might sometimes come from natural foods, but they are altered in some way after harvest. (They are "processed" or "refined.") Typically, the bran and germ are removed from the grain (leaving only the endosperm) which gives the grain a finer texture and longer shelf life.

What makes this problematic for the temple fueling system is that when the bran and germ are removed, so is the fiber, vitamins, and minerals that were in the bran and germ. These grains then become almost "empty calories."

This processing also changes the makeup of the food. The grain becomes a carbohydrate that "looks" like a complex carb but acts like a simple carb because it digests quickly.

These refined carbohydrates are a man-made fuel that the temple just isn't designed to use, in my opinion. The most common ones are white flour, white bread, white rice, pastries, sodas, packaged snacks, white sugar, refined syrups, some pasta, candies, and some breakfast cereals.

Foods that are labeled "enriched" are also considered refined carbohydrates. Because the grains were stripped of their nutrients and fiber during processing, companied sometimes add nutrients back in to the food to make up for what was lost. In other words, they are "enriched" with nutrients because they became deficient in nutrients during processing. The problem is, companies often add *synthetic* vitamins back into the food, which is not ideal. (I will talk much more about synthetic vitamins in later chapters.)

Gauging Fuel Efficiency

Refined carbohydrates can cause an immediate and drastic increase in blood sugar levels, followed by a drastic drop back to normal or below normal. If you were to chart it, it would look like that first (steep) hill on a rollercoaster that goes way up and then way down.

Complex carbs, on the other hand, digest slowly, so the increase and decrease are not as steep or dramatic. If you were to chart the digestion of complex carbs, it would look like a slow Sunday drive over a small gradual hill. To recap, refined carbs create a fast, intense, and stressful glucose response in the body (like a rollercoaster), whereas complex carbs create a steadier, less intense, non-stressful response in the body (like a Sunday drive).

Regarding fuel *efficiency*, it's important to aim for the Sunday drive—to choose carbohydrates that will not cause dramatic spikes and falls in blood sugar levels. As we talked about in the last chapter, these constant spikes and falls can lead to weight gain as well as many other serious health issues over time, including insulin resistance and hypoglycemia.

But how can you tell a rollercoaster carb from a Sunday drive carb? By using what's known as the glycemic index (GI). The GI Index is a measuring system that indicates what kind of glucose response a food will initiate in the body. Each food is ranked on a scale from 0-100. Foods low on the GI scale (45 and below) are typically complex carbs that contain fiber and protein, and so they release glucose slowly and steadily (Sunday drive). Foods high on the GI scale do not have as much fiber and protein, and so they release glucose rapidly (rollercoaster).

For example, a bowl of corn cereal ranks around 85 on the GI index, but a raw apple ranks around 34, even though both contain approximately 25 carbohydrates per serving. The cereal, though, is processed in a factory and stripped of most of its nutrients, so it creates a dramatic spike in blood sugar (rollercoaster). The apple, on the other hand, still contains all its natural fiber and protein, so it is digested slower and creates a less dramatic increase (Sunday drive).

Another example: mashed potatoes rank around 90 on the GI index, but chickpeas rank around 20, even though a serving of each contains approximately 30 carbohydrates. The reason: chickpeas are often just rinsed and canned, and then eaten raw, so they still contain their fiber and protein. Potatoes, on the other hand, are first peeled of their skin (which contains the fiber and protein), and then are boiled at high temperatures causing a loss of enzymes and nutrients. So, the end product is a rollercoaster carbohydrate high on the GI index. (The same can be true for the apple, though, if it is skinned and cooked at high temperatures to make applesauce. In that case, it will rank much higher on the GI index.)

Now, the GI scale is not a perfect system because you also need to take into consideration where the entire meal ranks on the scale. A high GI food like potatoes paired with protein-rich grilled salmon has a collectively lower ranking than just eating mashed potatoes by itself. But it's still higher than eating salmon with a side salad, instead of potatoes.

It's also important to consider where *your day* falls on the scale. Many people get stuck on what I call "the all-day rollercoaster." They eat white bread toast for breakfast, a white bread sandwich for lunch, and rice or dinner rolls for dinner. In between, that they have crackers, pretzels and chips for snacks, and soda and sugar-spiked coffee for beverages. Throughout the day their fueling system runs like a crazy thrill ride with fast, intense ups and downs... which explains why they're exhausted at the end of the day.

If this is you, friend, my advice is to get off the rollercoaster. Avoid high GI foods— especially while trying to rebuild the temple fueling system. But if there are times when you cannot avoid these foods, it is best to pair them with other protein or fiber-rich foods at least to slow digestion some. (Note: in the *Rebuilding Your Temple Workbook*, there is a detailed list of common carbohydrate foods and their GI ranking.)

Identifying Complex Carbs

If you are shopping and you don't have a GI index handy, there are other ways to discern good carbs and bad carbs. Carbohydrate fuel should come from foods that are closest to their natural form—the way you'd find them in nature—how the Architect designed them for temple fueling system.

For example, bread (and flour) should not be white. Most grains grown in nature are tan or brownish color. If it's white, that typically means the grain was processed and probably bleached. Also, it should be coarse in texture. Flours that are industrially refined are ground into a very fine powder, which yes, might make for a softer bread or cake, but they are digested quickly, and therefore will raise blood sugar levels quickly. This is what gives them a higher GI ranking.

Put simply: complex carbohydrates should be the first choice, and natural, simple carbs the second choice (unless you're getting ready to exercise and need a quicker fuel, then simple carbs like berries or orange slices might work better). Refined carbs should never be a choice at all, in my opinion. To identify which foods are which, though, you must read food labels and ingredient lists when you shop. You cannot always tell a good carb from the front of a package.

As I mentioned, the first thing you want to look for is fiber and protein. Unrefined whole grains that are complex carbohydrates will contain both of these. However, these still do not *guarantee* it is pure and unrefined. You also must read the ingredients list, not just the macronutrients.

Look for the word "whole" grain, which means that *all* parts of that grain are present. It means the bran, germ, and endosperm of the wheat kernel are "whole" and intact... and therefore, the grain is higher in vitamins, minerals, and fiber. If the word "whole" is not present, then the grain is probably refined in some way.

Also, words such as "enriched" and "degerminated" indicate that the grain has undergone processing of some kind.

And do not just quickly skim the front label looking for the words "whole grain." There is still much more to consider—like other ingredients and the _order_ of these ingredients. Typically, ingredients are listed in order of amount, meaning the first ingredient is the most plentiful ingredient. Every ingredient after that is present to a lesser degree.

So, let's say a bread label lists: "whole grain wheat flour, enriched white flour, and oat flour." This means that there is more whole grain wheat flour present than any other flour because it's listed first (even though it could be as little as 1% more). It also means there is more enriched white flour than there is oat flour. So, this food "could" be predominantly a complex carbohydrate because the first ingredient is a whole grain... but it's not guaranteed. The other two refined flours listed second and third could collectively outweigh the whole grain wheat flour which is listed first. This would make it a predominantly refined carbohydrate food.

This is especially true if multiple refined flours are listed first and only one whole grain flour is listed later in the list. If it's listed later in the list, it could contain as little as 2% of the whole grain. Therefore, do _not_ just look at the front of packages. Often a front label may claim (in big, bold letters) that the food contains "whole grains," but these whole grains are relatively useless if it is outweighed by copious amounts of refined flours which will inevitably cause a rollercoaster in your body.

That's not all. Even products that list _all_ whole grains in the ingredients can be unhealthy if they aren't organic and non-GMO. Why does this matter? Because, if the grains are not organic or non-GMO, they likely contain substantial amounts of pesticides. Multiple studies have clearly shown a correlation between pesticides and increased blood sugar, even diabetes. (1) I will talk much more about pesticides in later chapters.

Additionally, while organic "whole grains" are better than refined flours, there still might be an even healthier option—sprouted grains. Whole grains are like tiny seeds, but _sprouted_ grains are seeds that are soaked and have begun to grow or germinate (though aren't actual plants yet). It's like eating a little mini garden in your bread.

Several important things take place during the sprouting. First, most grains contain what are known as phytates (or phytic acid). Unfortunately, these phytates can block the absorption of minerals like iron, zinc, phosphorus, and magnesium. Phytates can also inhibit enzymes that are needed to break down the grain during digestion. But soaking grains, and allowing them to sprout, kills the phytic acid so the body can absorb more of the nutrients in the grain. Sprouting grains can also increase the fiber content of the grain and help with protein digestion.

A Caution About Wheat

So far, it may seem as though sprouted whole grain wheat is the healthiest, complex carbohydrate around. If you're a bread lover, you may be doing your happy dance. But don't get too excited. This type of wheat may be healthier than its counterparts, but that doesn't make it healthy for everyone.

The fact of the matter is: wheat has changed. Wheat today is _not_ the same wheat our grandparents ate. It has been crossbred over the last fifty years, and the new "hybrid strains" of wheat are genetically and biologically different than old or "ancient" wheat, plain and simple. In olden times, people ate wheat varieties like Emmer, Einkorn, and Kamut. Today nearly all commercial wheat is a shorter, "dwarf wheat" that produces not only high yield crops but also many health concerns.

First, certain wheat proteins today provoke an inflammatory immune response in the GI tract. This can weaken the lining of the gut wall (which is already thinner than your eyelid!) Gluten, specifically, stimulates the release of zonulin, which loosens the junctions between cells in the gut. (2) (3) This can allow undigested food particles to slip out of the intestines into the bloodstream.

When this happens, the immune system considers it a foreign substance (an invader), and it sends out red flags (antibodies) to find and destroy the gluten. Over time, this can develop into a wheat/gluten sensitivity, allergy, or even a serious autoimmune condition like Celiac Disease.

What's also alarming is that this new gluten looks a lot like various tissues in the body—especially thyroid tissue. So sometimes, the immune system can get confused. Since gluten and thyroid tissue look alike, some immune cells can end up attacking the thyroid by mistake, thinking it's gluten. It's a case of mistaken identity (also known as molecular mimicry), which can lead to other autoimmune diseases like Hashimoto's Disease. (I highly recommend a great article by Dr. Amy Meyers called "3 Important Reasons to Give Up Gluten if You Have an Autoimmune Disease" located here: https://www.amymyersmd.com/2018/04/3-reasons-give-up-gluten-autoimmune-disease/

Once upon a time, it was thought that wheat was just a concern for people who have a wheat allergy, Celiac Disease, or a genetic predisposition for it (if a family member has "issues with wheat"). But a 2006 study showed that another wheat protein—gliadin—activates zonulin too, regardless of whether you have the gene or not! (4) In other words, wheat can affect _anyone_, whether you have a family history or not.

Not convinced? Another study compared the effects of ancient Kamut wheat and modern wheat on healthy participants. Ancient Kamut caused a reduction in cholesterol, blood sugar, and inflammation compared to modern wheat, which in some cases increased it. (5) What's more, another study showed that ancient Einkorn caused significantly fewer reactions in celiac patients than modern gluten. (6) So the question is: is it all wheat or just new wheat that is problematic?

My belief: the Architect of your temple didn't design the fueling system to use this new wheat hybrid efficiently. But if you aren't willing to give it up just yet, then follow the strategy outlined here to choose the healthiest kind. Whole grain wheat flour is better than refined or enriched wheat flour. But _organic_ whole wheat is even better than regular whole wheat. Organic _sprouted_ wheat is better than even organic whole grain wheat. And ancient wheat is better than sprouted modern wheat. Confused? Here's how it looks from best to worst:

1. Organic ancient grains
2. Organic sprouted wheat
3. Organic whole grain wheat
4. Non-organic whole grain wheat
5. Refined or enriched wheat

Now, that's the general order. However, when we are talking about rebuilding your temple, I don't think that picking a fuel from the low end of the totem pole is going to get the job done. This is especially true if you have an autoimmune disease, thyroid issues, leaky gut syndrome (or any gut issues, actually), or if you even _suspect_ you (or anyone in your family) has these issues.

My professional recommendation: Ditch. The. Wheat. Take the same principles outlined here and apply them to other, gluten-free grains. Look for bread with organic, gluten-free ancient grains (preferably sprouted) like amaranth, buckwheat, millet, sorghum, and teff. Or begin a grain-free paleo diet, using flours such as almond and coconut. But whatever you do, do _not_ choose gluten-free grains like rice and corn that are not organic or non-GMO verified. They are just as harmful as non-organic wheat. (Again, I will talk much more about GMOs later on.)

If you do _not_ have any of the above issues (or a family history of these issues), and you do not want to give up wheat at this time, then I _strongly_ advise you to at least limit the quantity of it—and by "limit" I mean only eating wheat at one meal a day. That means if you have wheat toast for breakfast, then do not to have a sandwich at lunch or pasta at dinner.

If you're not quite sure whether you or someone in your family has an autoimmune disease, check the list at the link below. There are more than 100 classified autoimmune diseases currently, with 40 more being studied.

http://autoimmunesociety.org/diseases-disorders/

Replace Don't Erase

Some of you may be feeling disappointed or overwhelmed by my suggestion to ditch the wheat. I'm assuming it wasn't what you wanted to hear. I get it. I do. But, I'm not going to sugar-coat things. I'm going to be straight with you throughout this rebuild because I have your best interest at heart. I want this rebuild to work for you. As I said at the beginning, I'm going to ask you to do some hard things here. You have to be willing to change your habits if you want to see a change in your temple.

Now, this doesn't mean you have to suffer a life of deprivation, starvation, and misery. No, no NOOOO. If you live like that when it comes to food, then you will ultimately fail. Plain and simple.

My philosophy when I coach clients is to "replace, not erase." What I mean by that is, don't erase everything from your diet. Try to find healthy replacements for your unhealthy favorites. And please understand that you _can_ reprogram your taste buds. You might not think so now, but try to remember, you are in the "rebuilding" stages. You are "under construction." This is not how you're going to be forever.

A lot of times, we look at the unhealthy things about us (like our taste buds), and we assume that's "how we're made." We tell ourselves things like, "I'm just a carb addict." Or "I'm just a glutton." Or "I'm just a healthy eater." But that's not necessarily how we're _made_, that's just how we _became_ after years of eating.

What you crave now does not have to be what you will crave for the rest of your life. Trust me. I've seen it time and time again with myself and many, _many_ clients. For example, one client used to crave pastries nearly to the point of addiction. Now she craves things like lettuce and cucumbers. Another client didn't think he could ever give up his bowl of late-night ice cream. Not only did he give it up, he now thinks ketchup is too sweet for his burger. YOUR TASTE BUDS CAN CHANGE— that is, if you give them a chance by exposing them to other things, eliminating the problem foods, and giving the body what it needs when you are craving something specific. (There's a chart of what common cravings mean in the _Rebuilding Your Temple Workbook_.)

Now, let's talk about healthy replacements. We already went over bread and choosing different grains. Now let's discuss other types of carbs.

Pasta

Most boxed pasta is made with "enriched" wheat flour (meaning it was stripped and then enriched later with vitamins to make up for what was lost). So how do you replace pasta? Start reading labels and search for one that is NOT enriched. Use the same strategy as you do when choosing grains: look for whole grain, organic, non-GMO, fiber, and protein.

Another (better) option is to use a vegetable spiralizer and make organic zucchini noodles. No, it's not the same as wheat pasta. Yes, it has a different taste and texture. But it's still very appetizing—and it's a veggie, so it's full of fiber, vitamins, phytonutrients and antioxidants that contribute positively to overall health. (This is the ultimate goal, after all, right?) Plus, if you want to reprogram your taste buds, you need to expose them to new things.

Another option is to switch to pasta made from non-grains such as spinach, chickpeas, black beans, and red lentils. But read the ingredients list to make sure it's 100% non-grains. The first ingredient should *not* be enriched flour with non-grains listed lower on the label.

Rice

White rice has a high GI ranking of about 75. Not only that, white rice is milled, and the bran removed (making it a white color). This decreases the fiber content and nutritional value. So, does that mean you should switch to brown rice? Well, not necessarily. Brown rice has more nutrients and fiber, yes, but it is much higher in phytic acid as well as arsenic. (I will talk more about this in later chapters.)

I recommend replacing grain rice with cauli-rice! I take a head of cauliflower, break it apart, put it in a blender or food processor, and turn it on! Voila! Rice! You can sauté it with a tablespoon of butter (or a few beaten eggs if you want a thicker/chunkier consistency). And, yes, it tastes different than actual rice, but it's very versatile, and the texture holds up well as a rice substitute in many recipes.

Baked Goods

Some of you love your baked goods and can't imagine living life without them… Yeah, I get it. That was me, too. The good news is you don't have to. You just have to change the way you make them by substituting wheat flour for grain-free or gluten-free flours (like almond flour and coconut flour). The internet is full of very tasty recipes.

If you're reading these replacement ideas and you're thinking there is no possible way you're going to like them, or if you're not willing to even try them, then let me say this: you cannot continue to do the same things over and over again and expect different results. If you want to rebuild, to see and feel a change in your temple, then you have to be willing to change your diet.

Fiber

As I said, one of the things that makes a complex carbohydrate "complex" is its fiber content. When fiber is digested, the body handles it differently than it does other carbohydrates. Part of the fiber goes through the digestive system without breaking down at all. This is important for a couple of reasons.

One, fiber doesn't cause a spike in blood sugar levels or trigger an insulin release like other carbs do, so they're essentially "free" carbs when it comes to glucose balance. For this reason, if you want to determine how many *actual*, glucose-affecting carbs (a.k.a. "net" carbs) are in a food, subtract the number of fibers from the number of total carbs. For example, a slice of bread that has 12 carbohydrates and five fibers really only has seven net carbs per slice (12 total carbs - 5 fibers = 7 net carbs).

What's more, both types of fiber (soluble and insoluble) help to keep bowels regular. Soluble fiber dissolves in water, forming a gel, so it helps water stay in the stool, making it softer and easier to pass. Insoluble fiber does not dissolve in water, so it adds bulk to the stool, making the colon feel full so that it begins the elimination process.

Many high fiber foods contain both soluble and insoluble fiber, but they are usually higher in one than the other. Some of the top sources of bulk-forming insoluble fiber are high-carbohydrate foods like wheat and other whole grains, lentils, and beans. They are not keto-friendly, obviously, so keep that in mind if you decide to switch fuels. Some *low* carb options that are high in insoluble fiber include flaxseed, chia seeds, leafy greens, broccoli, cauliflower, and celery... these _are_ keto-friendly.

Foods with water-absorbing soluble fiber include apples, pears, brussels sprouts, oats, rye, and barley (but they are not keto-friendly). Nuts, psyllium (or psyllium husk), carrots, onions, and chicory root are high in soluble fiber and low in carbs (so they are keto-friendly).

Typically, adult women should try to get at least 25 grams of fiber daily, and men should try for 35 grams. This could be higher for those with high cholesterol or who are at risk for heart disease, as studies have shown that soluble fiber can lower both total cholesterol and LDL cholesterol. (7) Other studies show greater fiber intake can substantially reduce the risk of coronary heart disease, and particularly coronary death. (8)

Getting this much fiber every day may seem like a difficult task for some (especially if you go keto), but it's not impossible. It just requires planning and diligence. Here are a couple of ways to incorporate more fiber into your diet:

1. Eat a big garden salad at least once every single day.
2. Add chia seeds, hemp seeds, and flaxseed to your smoothies.
3. Add psyllium husk to your homemade baked goods.
4. Have raw veggies (broccoli, celery, cauliflower) with a homemade dip as your snack.

Please note: if you aren't used to eating this much fiber, _ease_ into it. Do not start with the recommended 25-35 grams/day as it can make you gassy if your system isn't used to it.

Sugars

We've already talked about complex and refined carbs, and how they affect blood sugar levels. Now let's talk about simple carbs, aka natural sugars. Sugars found in fruits and dairy products are healthy carbohydrates. Yes, they cause a more immediate rise in blood sugar than complex carbs do, but this can be tempered with the fiber in the fruit skin or the protein in the milk. These sugars are not harmful to glucose levels in most cases.

This is completely different from white sugar, brown sugar, and other processed sweeteners. Yes, regular table sugar has a lower GI rating than white rice, but that does _not_ mean sugar is good for you. No, no, no, no. Here are some things you should know about sugar:

Sugar stresses the Liver

Almost all "added sugars" (including table sugar, even organic cane sugar) contain substantial amounts of fructose. Fructose goes straight to the liver to be processed. If it's fructose from a piece of fruit, it is metabolized slowly because, as I said, it contains fiber from the fruit skin and fruit flesh (so it's not harmful). But, if it is fructose that has been extracted from the fiber source, and then added to other foods as a sweetener, then it is metabolized very quickly... just like alcohol, actually.

The other problem is, the liver is limited in how much fructose it can metabolize at one time. Excess fructose (anything more than the storing limit), is then metabolized into fat, which is stored in the liver. This can lead to what is known as non-alcoholic fatty liver disease (NAFLD), fat build-up in the liver, and non-alcoholic steatohepatitis (NASH), liver inflammation and scarring. This is a serious condition as approximately one-quarter of those with NASH develop liver cirrhosis, which can require a liver transplant. (9)

According to sugarscience.org, *"Since 1980, the incidence of NAFLD and NASH has doubled along with the rise of fructose consumption. Approximately 6 million individuals in the United States are estimated to have progressed to NASH and some 600,000 to NASH-related cirrhosis... Most people with NASH also have Type II diabetes."* (10)

Sugar increases Cholesterol and Triglycerides

According to Dr. Lustig from sugarscience.org, the liver can safely metabolize only about six teaspoons of added sugar per day. The excess that is metabolized into fat is then released into the bloodstream. This is what causes high triglycerides, high cholesterol, and high blood pressure. (11)

What's more, a study of more than 40,000 people published in JAMA Internal Medicine shows that those with the highest sugar intake had a 400% increase in their risk of heart attacks compared to those with the lowest intakes! And just one 20-ounce soda can increase your risk of a heart attack by about 30%. (12)

Sugar is Addictive

To make matters worse, sugar can create an addictive response in the brain (13) (14). When you eat sugar, you receive a dopamine signal and experience pleasure, which causes you to consume more sugar. The problem is, with prolonged exposure, the signal gets weaker. So, you have to consume more sugar to get the same pleasurable effect — this can lead to sugar tolerance. If you eliminate sugar, then, you can experience withdrawal. Tolerance and withdrawal are the two main components of addiction.

What's more, animal studies have shown that intense sweetness can surpass even a cocaine reward in the brain. (12) According to Doctor Mark Hyman, sugar is eight times as addictive as cocaine. Sugar has been found to activate not just one, but *many* areas of the nucleus accumbens (the brain region that controls addiction). (15)

Too Much Sugar Can Lead to Vitamin and Mineral Deficiencies

Sugar and vitamin C use the same transporters to reach cells. So basically, more sugar in the bloodstream can equate to decreased vitamin C absorption. Decreased vitamin C absorption can lead to weakened immunity, premature aging (vitamin C is needed for collagen synthesis), inflammation, and impaired neurotransmitter synthesis.

Sugar also increases enzymes that destroy vitamin D and decreases enzymes needed to make vitamin D. So, excess sugar can lead to vitamin D deficiency too.

Sugar raises blood sugar levels, thereby raising insulin levels, and raised insulin causes the body to eliminate magnesium (which the body needs for more than 300 biochemical processes). So, excess sugar can also lead to magnesium deficiency.

Sugar also hinders chromium absorption, which can lead to a chromium deficiency (and chromium is an *essential* trace mineral, meaning the body NEEDS chromium in trace amounts in order to operate properly).

What's more, because sugar can lead to vitamin D and vitamin C deficiencies (which are both needed for calcium absorption), excess sugar also can also lead to calcium deficiency.

As you can see, sugar can have a huge impact on multiple areas of the body, not just on blood sugar. That's why one of the single, most beneficial things you can do for your weight and your overall health is to give up sugar. I absolutely cannot stress this enough.

Sweeteners:

Some of you may now be wondering about sweeteners such as Splenda®, Nutra Sweet®, or Equal®. Perhaps you're thinking of switching to these sugar-free alternatives now that I've vilified sugar. But, hold on for just a minute. My advice is to stay far (FAR) away from these too.

The reasons are many, but I'll list a few important ones. Let's start with Aspartame (NutraSweet® and Equal®). Aspartame is the most widely used sweetener in the world. It has zero calories and tastes 200 times sweeter than sugar, but it breaks down into phenylalanine and aspartic acid (which act as neurotoxins when absorbed too quickly). It also breaks down into methanol (which is wood alcohol found in antifreeze) and is then oxidized into formaldehyde in various tissues. Yes, formaldehyde... you know, the fluid that morticians use for embalming. Yummy.

Studies show aspartame causes migraines, especially in youth (16), but this is just one of the more than 90 reported side effects! It also affects DNA (especially in the mitochondria), damages the structure of the sciatic nerve, (17) causes weight gain, (18) and neurophysiological symptoms such as learning difficulty, seizures, migraines, irritable moods, anxiety, depression, and insomnia. (19)

Aspartame is hard to avoid, though, because it's found in more than 6000 products--things like "diet" foods, frozen desserts, gelatins, puddings, fillings, nutrition bars, chewing gum, soda, powdered soft drinks, tabletop sweeteners, and yogurt. Even sugar-free pharmaceuticals like cough drops contain aspartame. The only way to avoid it is to read labels and eat real food.

Sucralose

Now let's talk about Splenda, aka Sucralose. Sucralose is said to be 600 times sweeter than table sugar without the calories. The claim is that sucralose comes from sugar, so it's a more natural non-calorie sweetener—and yes, it does start from a sugar (sucrose) molecule. But then three chlorine molecules are added to the sugar molecule (yes, *chlorine*). This changes the chemical structure drastically. In fact, Dr. Mercola says, chemically, "Splenda is actually more similar to DDT than sugar." (20)

The Architect did not design the temple of the human body to use a "sugar" like this. It is not properly metabolized. This is evident through recent studies which show sucralose consumption leads to increased insulin secretion, elevated glucose levels, reduced glucagon secretion, delayed gastric emptying, altered sweet taste receptors, a 50% reduction in good gut flora, induced DNA damage, and increased risk for weight gain as well as the development of diabetes. (21)

What's more, cooking with sucralose at high temperatures can generate chloropropanols, a potentially toxic class of compounds. (21)

Plain and simple, it's advisable to stay far away from saccharin, aspartame, sucralose, acesulfame K, and neotame.

High Fructose Corn Syrup

I would be remiss if I didn't also talk about another harmful sweetener called high fructose corn syrup. High Fructose Corn Syrup (and "corn syrup") are synthetic food ingredients. Like other artificial sweeteners, the temple of the body does not know what to do with these or how to digest them. This form of fructose can confuse the brain, affect hunger hormones, and increase appetite. (22)

Research also shows a connection between high fructose corn syrup and disrupted stress hormones, fat accumulation, reduced glucose tolerance, insulin resistance, higher triglycerides, and cholesterol, (23) and increased blood pressure. (24) High doses of free fructose have even been proven to punch holes in the intestinal lining. (25)

What's more, it's been reported that nearly half of all tested samples of commercial high-fructose corn syrup contained mercury. (24) In fact, some estimate it contains up to 570 micrograms of mercury per gram.

Again, if you want to avoid this sweetener (which you should), you're going to have to be diligent and read labels as you shop.

Safe Sweeteners

So now the big question is, what sweeteners ARE safe? My top two recommendations are Stevia and Monk Fruit. Stevia is a very sweet herb (200 times sweeter than sugar) that does not raise blood glucose levels. However, it is part of the ragweed family and can be problematic for those with a ragweed allergy. Also, some powdered forms of Stevia can undergo processing, such as bleaching. They also may have added ingredients such as maltodextrin (from corn), so it is important to choose a reputable brand that is non-GMO verified.

Another, and perhaps even better sweetener, is monk fruit. Monk fruit contains a significant amount of antioxidants to fight free radicals; it is 300-400 times sweeter than sugar but does not have any calories or effect on blood sugar levels. It also acts as an antihistamine and is anti-inflammatory. Monk fruit is also sold in liquid and powder form.

Juice

While we are on the subject of fructose, let's talk about juice for a minute. Many people think that just because it's labeled FRUIT juice, it's healthy. But, that's not necessarily the case. Juices that are mostly made of corn syrup and food dye are to be avoided at all cost, in my opinion. The same goes for juices that are labeled "low sugar," because they are likely sweetened with sucralose, which we've already discussed.

Other juices that list "fruit juice concentrate" as the main ingredient should also be avoided because it is primarily processed fructose. Even some juices made from 100% fruit, have been found to have higher fructose concentrations than those made with high fructose corn syrup. (27)

I've already talked about the problems that excess fructose can create in the liver. But it also plays a direct role in the risk for metabolic disease, (27) increased appetite, (28) and the proliferation of cancer cells. (29)

What's more, fructose cannot be used for energy by cells. It has to be converted into a usable form first, which can take several hours. Many harmful bacteria in the gut <u>can</u> use it for energy, though, causing a bacterial overgrowth (which I will talk about extensively in later chapters).

Now, back to juice. You might argue that there are vitamins in fruit juice, so it's good for you... right? Wrong. Bottled juice is pasteurized. Pasteurization is the process of heating food to kill any bad bacteria, so it will be safe to eat. But, bacteria are not all that pasteurization kills.

Many of the vitamins in the fruit are also destroyed in the heating process. In fact, ascorbic acid (vitamin C) is especially sensitive to heat and is lost the most (which is ironic because most people drink fruit juice specifically for vitamin C). Not to mention, fruit juice concentrate is created from a heating process, so pasteurized juice made from concentrate can potentially be heated twice before it hits shelves. Because of all this processing, synthetic vitamins are often added back into the juice (it is "fortified") to make up for the loss.

The bottom line is, juice is not a health-food, unless it is fresh-squeezed in your kitchen. Instead, we should develop a taste for WATER which is needed by every cell in the body. If you need to flavor it because you aren't used to it yet, try squeezing a lemon in the water and add liquid Stevia for lemonade. Or buy a juicer and make it yourself with pulp for fiber.

References

1. http://www.diabetesandenvironment.org/home/contam/pesticides
2. https://www.ncbi.nlm.nih.gov/pmc/articles/PMC5084031/
3. https://www.ncbi.nlm.nih.gov/pmc/articles/PMC3384703/
4. https://www.researchgate.net/profile/Tarcisio_Not/publication/7144746_Gliadin_zonulin_and_gut_permeability_Effects_on_celiac_and_non-celiac_intestinal_mucosa_and_intestinal_cell_lines/links/09e41506495e140c7d000000/Gliadin-zonulin-and-gut-permeability-Effects-on-celiac-and-non-celiac-intestinal-mucosa-and-intestinal-cell-lines.pdf
5. https://www.ncbi.nlm.nih.gov/pubmed/23299714
6. https://www.ncbi.nlm.nih.gov/pmc/articles/PMC3664588/
7. circ.ahajournals.org/content/94/11/2720
8. https://academic.oup.com/ajcn/article/69/1/30/4694117
9. https://www.ncbi.nlm.nih.gov/pubmed/2295475
10. sugarscience.ucsf.edu/the-toxic-truth/#.W0dQvvZFzIU
11. https://jamanetwork.com/journals/jamainternalmedicine/fullarticle/1819573
12. https://www.ncbi.nlm.nih.gov/pmc/articles/PMC2235907/
13. https://academic.oup.com/ajcn/article/98/3/641/4577039
14. https://www.ncbi.nlm.nih.gov/pmc/articles/PMC1931610/
15. https://drhyman.com/blog/2013/06/27/5-clues-you-are-addicted-to-sugar/
16. https://www.ncbi.nlm.nih.gov/pubmed/18627677
17. https://www.ncbi.nlm.nih.gov/pmc/articles/PMC6014252/

18. https://www.ncbi.nlm.nih.gov/pmc/articles/PMC2892765/
19. https://www.ncbinlm.nih.gov/pubmed/28198207
20. https://articles.mercola.com/sites/articles/archive/2011/04/26/major-media-finally-exposes-splendas-lies.aspx
21. https://www.ncbi.nlm.nih.gov/pmc/articles/PMC3856475/
22. https://www.ncbi.nlm.nih.gov/pubmed/18627777/
23. https://www.ncbi.nlm.nih.gov/pmc/articles/PMC3522469/
24. https://www.ncbi.nlm.nih.gov/pmc/articles/PMC3139867/
25. https://www.huffingtonpost.com/dr-mark-hyman/high-fructose-corn-syrup-dangers_b_861913.html
26. www.washingtonpost.com/wp-dyn/content/article/2009/01/26/AR2009012601831.html?noredirect=on
27. https://www.ncbi.nlm.nih.gov/pubmed/23594708
28. https://www.ncbi.nlm.nih.gov/pubmed/23280226
29. cancerres.aacrjournals.org/content/70/15/6368

Chapter 3: Installing a Thermostat

If you think of a house again, it can use various sources of energy such as electricity, propane, natural gas, etc. But, for the house to remain at a steady temperature (and for the furnace/fueling system to not be overworked), you have to install a thermostat which determines how much fuel should be used, and at what times it should be used.

Such is the case for the temple of the body, too. Choosing the right kind of fuel (complex carbs or healthy fats) is only part of the equation. The other part is choosing is how much fuel is needed and when it's needed. To do this, we need a "temple thermostat" that can gauge our needs as well as our intake of macronutrients (macros) such as calories, fat, carbs, and protein. You can do this digitally by installing a macro tracking app on your smartphone, or manually by using a tracking worksheet (which can be found in the *Rebuilding Your Temple Workbook*).

I know. I know. Some of you already aren't happy about the idea of tracking what you eat. I get it. I do. It sounds like a pain. And some other health professionals will disagree with me on this. They will say, "Just eat real food, and you will be fine." However, I've seen this to be false with many clients (even myself). Some people are eating way too much "real food," and others are not eating enough, so they do not see results.

Think about it. What if someone told you they didn't need a thermostat for their house? You'd say they were nuts. Believe me when I say, it's just as nuts not to track your fuel when you first start on this rebuild. Trust me.

You might think, "I'll just eat when I'm hungry, and I'll stop eating when I'm full," but that's like manually using a furnace. It's not going to work *efficiently*, which is our primary goal. First, your appetite right now could be controlled by too many unreliable factors—irregular hunger hormones, blood sugar imbalances, harmful gut bacteria. With these issues present, your appetite simply cannot accurately tell you when you *really* need to eat and how much you need.

This is not just for those who want to lose weight, either. It's for those who want to be healthy, who want to be assured they are getting enough protein, healthy fats, quality carbohydrates, fiber, and water. To be honest, most people who start rebuilding haven't been getting enough of one or more of their macros (or perhaps are getting too much), so this is an important training exercise.

This is a process that will help you "see" food differently. The goal is to retrain the brain to see food in _numbers_. Instead of seeing just a small pastry, we need to see 100 carbs, 65 sugars, and 30 fats. We need to see that in that "little" pastry is a whole day's worth (or at least a half of a day's worth) of total carbs and fats.

Often, we see food as just meals and snacks. You might look at your day and think, "I only ate two meals and one snack today. Why can't I lose weight?" But it's crucial to see snacks and meals in their true form, broken down in numbers of macronutrients. Those "two" meals and that "one" snack might have been 3,000 calories with 50% coming from refined carbohydrates. Or those "two" meals might have been severely lacking in protein and fiber, which contributed to rollercoaster blood sugars.

The other reason this is important is that, if you aren't tracking, you're snacking. It's not uncommon to pick at "little" snacks here and there throughout the day. They seem so insignificant that you barely realize you've done it. But, these are part of the energy supply. They affect the fueling system, and they do add up... especially when they are fat calories.

Using a tracking method (or a temple thermostat) helps provide the temple with a steady supply of fuel, but only fuel that is actually needed for energy (so that excess fuel is not stored as fat). This is enormously important at the beginning of the rebuild.

Types of Thermostats

If you have a smartphone, the easiest way to track your macros is to use an app. There are many different ones to choose from. (I use an app called MyMacros+.) An app allows you to keep track of the calories, fat, carbs, protein, and fiber you consume with every meal and snack. This running tally helps you see how close or far away you are from reaching your daily maximum.

If you are close to your daily max at 11 A.M., then you know you need to slow down the fuel supply for the rest of the day (and eat a smaller breakfast the next day.) If you are still a long way off at dinner, you know you can eat a hearty dinner without the guilt (and probably eat a little earlier in the day tomorrow).

With an app like My Macros+, you can search through hundreds of foods that already have the macros entered, so you don't have to type everything in. It also has a barcode scanner, too. You simply scan the barcode on the food packaging with your phone camera, and the numbers are automatically entered. It also allows you to input favorite or custom recipes, reuse recent foods, and set goals to track weight loss or weight gain.

If you do not have a smartphone, or if you are not very "technical" and do not use apps, there is a worksheet you can use in the *Rebuilding Your Temple Workbook*. It is a similar process where you keep a running tally of macros throughout the day, but everything will need to be written out manually. You can keep these worksheets in a 3-ring binder or keep one in your daily planner—somewhere convenient where you will have access to it throughout the day.

Calculating Fuel

Before you can "set your thermostat" (before you can set up your macro tracker) you will need to determine how *much* fuel you actually need. In other words, you need to figure out how many calories you should consume each day. The standard 2,000 calorie diet does not work for everyone. Every temple is drastically different with different genders, ages, jobs, exercise regimens, etc. Therefore, the amount of fuel needed is different for everyone too. A 5' 1" sedentary adult with a desk job, who does not exercise, does not need as many calories (as much fuel) as a 6' 3" construction worker, who works out intensely five days a week after work.

To calculate your unique numbers, go to www.RebuildingYourTemple.com and click "Macro Calculator." Type in your personal information (height, weight, age, etc.) and the calculator will tell you how many calories you need each day to reach your goals. You can also do this manually, using the worksheet in the *Rebuilding Your Temple Workbook*.

Converting to Macros

Once you have determined how many calories you need each day, you will need to convert those calories into grams of protein, fat, and carbs. These are called your macronutrients, or "macros" for short. These calculations will differ significantly depending on your goals, health issues, and the type of fuel you wish to use (if you're keto or using glucose).

To calculate your macros, enter your "daily calories" number from above into the calculations below. Choose only ONE of the below calculations, and discuss these calculations with your doctor or dietician to ensure they are safe for you BEFORE implementing them. The calculations below are only a general guideline used by some people. It is also advised that you use the *Rebuilding Your Temple Workbook* to record this relevant information.

1.) The Standard Keto Diet

According to experts, a standard ketogenic diet should contain a low amount of carbohydrates (around 5-10%), with moderate amounts of lean protein (15-20%) and high amounts of healthy fats, which is the body's primary fuel (70-80%). Use the below calculations to determine your unique numbers. Again, discuss these calculations with your doctor or dietician BEFORE implementing them.

- Calculate daily grams of fat: [daily calories x .80] ÷ 9 = maximum daily fat intake
- Calculate daily grams of protein: [daily calories x .15] ÷ 4 = maximum daily protein intake
- Calculate daily grams of carbohydrate: [daily calories x .05] ÷ 4 = maximum daily carb intake

2.) Standard Glucose Diet

According to experts, a standard glucose diet for non-sedentary, exercising adults should contain a higher amount of carbohydrates (40-50%), which is the body's primary fuel. It should have plenty of fiber (25 grams for women and 35 grams for men). And it should contain a moderate amount of lean protein (20-30%) and healthy fat (20-30%). Use the below calculations to determine your unique numbers. Extreme or intense exercise regimens could require more carbohydrates (50-65%). Conversely, sedentary adults who do *not* exercise might need fewer carbohydrates (25-30%). Again, discuss these calculations with your doctor or dietician BEFORE implementing them.

- Calculate daily grams of fat: [daily calories x .30] ÷ 9 = maximum daily fat intake

- Calculate daily grams of protein: [daily calories x .25] ÷ 4 = maximum daily protein intake
- Calculate daily grams of carbohydrate: [daily calories x .45] ÷ 4 = maximum daily carb intake

Other Variations

Macros That May Assist Thyroid Function

The inactive thyroid hormone, T4, is converted into the active form, T3, in the liver and in muscle tissue (which depends on protein). Protein also transports thyroid hormones throughout your body once it is converted, and it helps stabilize rollercoaster blood sugars (which is essential for thyroid health). Therefore, some people with thyroid issues benefit from a high protein, liver-detoxifying, low-GI diet. This strategy contains a moderate amount of complex, wheat-free, non-grain carbohydrates (40%), higher amounts of lean protein (up to 30%), and moderate amounts of healthy fats (30%). Again, discuss these calculations with your doctor or dietician BEFORE implementing them.

Macros to Build Lean Muscle and Improve Metabolism

Protein has a thermic effect, which means your body creates heat during digestion and uses more calories in the digestive process (about 25% of protein calories are burned during digestion). So, eating more protein can potentially speed up metabolism in some people. (We will talk much more about this in later chapters.) Additionally, protein helps builds muscle, which also increases the metabolic rate.

Therefore, some people who want to build lean muscle and improve their metabolism benefit from a diet relatively high in protein (30-40%), with moderate fat and carbohydrate intake (25-30%). Use the below calculations to determine your unique numbers. *Note: for those who have a larger build and have a calorie allotment above 2200 calories/day, 30-40% protein may be difficult to achieve and difficult to digest (especially at the beginning). It may be better to start with a goal of 100-120 grams. Again, discuss these calculations with your doctor or dietician BEFORE implementing them.*

Macros to Help Balance Stress Hormones

Carbohydrates raise glucose and thereby, insulin. Insulin then pushes down the level of the stress hormone, cortisol. Therefore, some people who are trying to balance stress hormones benefit from a diet with moderate amounts of carbohydrates. Some also benefit from a moderate amount of protein because too much cortisol can potentially break down muscle tissue. However, it's a fine line because too much protein can reduce the calming neurotransmitter, GABA. A stress-friendly diet might also contain moderate amounts of healthy fats, such as omega 3 fatty acids because they have been shown to reduce cortisol levels too. (We will talk much more about omegas and cortisol in later chapters). Timing of these macros is also important (see "Thermostat Scheduling" below).

Thermostat Scheduling

Many home thermostats have scheduling capabilities, like an auto-schedule, basic schedule, or a pre-programmed schedule. Schedules help lower fueling costs and save energy. You don't want your furnace running overtime keeping your home warm while everyone is away at work and school. This is fuel wasting. However, you _do_ want the house to be warm when everyone comes home. So, this would require a schedule that starts to decrease fuel use when everyone leaves and increase it before everyone comes home from work/school.

Such is the case with the temple thermostat also. It's important to schedule your fuel for when it is needed most. Taking in calories when they are not needed could lead to fat storage as we have already discussed. Not only that, certain health issues require a specific macro schedule to use fuel efficiently.

Discuss the below fuel schedules with your doctor to determine if one is right for you.

The Stress Schedule

Those with chronic stress issues may need to eat in a way that assists their circadian rhythm—the body's natural sleep/wake cycle. Around 3:00 A.M., a healthy body starts to increase cortisol production to help you wake up and feel energized. About one hour after you wake up, cortisol levels should peak and be at their highest of the day. This is a good thing because it helps you "get going."

As the day goes on, though, these levels should drop steadily. You should have a medium amount of cortisol around lunchtime, and lower cortisol in the evening (so you can wind down and fall asleep).

Unfortunately, some people have a dysregulated circadian rhythm. What that means is they don't produce the right amount of cortisol at the right time of day. They either have too much cortisol production all day long, and it never lowers like it should. Or, they have low cortisol (fatigue) in the morning and higher cortisol (energy) in the evening. This is often why some people get a "second wind" after dinner and have difficulty falling asleep at night. Some people even have a cortisol peak in the middle of the night, so they wake up and can't fall back to sleep. For people with a dysregulated circadian rhythm, the macro _schedule_ is just as important as the type and amount of macros eaten, because food can either help or hurt cortisol balance and the rhythm.

As I mentioned above, carbohydrates increase blood sugar and insulin, which helps lower cortisol. Therefore, some people who are struggling with too much cortisol at night, find it beneficial to eat the majority of their carbs (complex carbs) at dinner. In the morning, they find a low-carb, high-protein and fat breakfast is more beneficial. This allows their cortisol to remain high/peaked in the morning, and it helps keep blood sugars and insulin steady.

Moderate amounts of healthy carbs at lunch then help start to lower cortisol. This can help reset the body's cortisol schedule to a healthier rhythm. The same philosophy can be applied during acute instances of stress. When cortisol increases due to a stressful moment or a stressful event, eating healthy carbohydrates during that stress can sometimes help lower cortisol and lessen the negative effects of stress (especially for those who are stress eaters).

Again, discuss this with your doctor or dietician BEFORE implementing a new diet or schedule.

The Blood Sugar Schedule

Some people who struggle with low blood sugars (hypoglycemia) benefit most from a diet with moderate amounts of carbohydrates that spread out throughout the day. Eating small balanced meals (with protein, fiber, fat, and carbs) every 2-3 hours is often most helpful.

On the other hand, some people with high blood sugars (hyperglycemia), benefit most from a ketogenic diet, or a low-to-moderate carbohydrate diet where carbs are spaced out throughout the day. Again, eating protein and fiber at every meal helps stabilize rollercoaster glucose levels. That being said, if you have blood sugar imbalances of any kind it is imperative to discuss your diet/schedule with your doctor before making any changes.

The Exercise Schedule

Another thing to take into consideration when scheduling your macros is exercise. It is vital to make sure you have enough fuel to sustain the body's energy needs. This can be done in three phases. Discuss these phases with your doctor before implementing them.

Phase 1

Non-keto rebuilders often consume slow-digesting, complex carbs that contain fiber and protein 2-3 hours before the workout. Eating protein and complex carbs too close to a workout could result in stomach upset as the body tries to digest the food while exercising. But eating these well enough in advance ensures the nutrients are readily available during the workout. It's important not to neglect protein in phase 1. Protein helps slow digestion and contains nitrogen molecules, which are needed to reach an anabolic state (when the body builds and repairs muscle tissue). Endurance athletes can eat a substantial amount of complex carbohydrates even up to 12 hours before their workout as the body can store up to 2,000 calories of glucose as glycogen. This will help sustain them for longer so that they do not "hit a wall" during the workout or race.

Phase 2

A few fast-acting, *simple* carbohydrates (like oranges) can then be eaten 20-30 minutes before exercise. These do not require much digestive work but will be an immediate source of fuel for the workout (they won't go to storage). Both Phase 1 and Phase 2 are important because, if during a high-intensity workout, you deplete your glycogen stores (the stored carbs in your muscles), your body will start to use your muscle as its next source of energy. Endurance athletes might benefit from higher amounts of fruit or even glucose gels to provide enough immediate fuel.

Phase 3

During exercise, muscle proteins break down. You might think, *"wait, this is the exact opposite of what I'm going for."* But after the workout, your body goes through what's called muscle protein synthesis, where it removes or repairs these damaged proteins and builds new, stronger, denser ones. So, if you are trying to build muscle (whether bulking or just toning), this only happens when the rate of muscle protein synthesis is higher than the rate of muscle protein breakdown (when you're building new ones more than breaking down old ones). And remember, protein synthesis happens *after* the workout. Therefore, post-workout food choices are every bit as important as pre-workout ones.

After a workout, it's vital to consume a generous amount of protein to help transport protein to the muscle for repair. Whey protein is one of the most quickly absorbed proteins, so it is an optimal post-workout choice. (I will talk much more about the different kinds of proteins in later chapters.) You will also want to eat a good amount of slow-digesting complex carbohydrates to replenish glycogen stores. It's important to note that the carbs and sugar found in fruit do _not_ replenish glycogen stores, so fruit is not an efficient fuel after exercise.

Exercise and Keto

Because a ketogenic diet is a low-carb diet, the body typically doesn't have enough carbs to serve as muscle glycogen. But it isn't necessary. Glycogen is stored carbohydrate fuel. In ketosis, the body runs on a different fuel. The problem is until you are keto-adapted, your body may still be in the habit of looking for glycogen during exercise. So, there may be a transition period you have to contend with.

If you plan to exercise more than three days a week or exercise at a high-intensity level in ketosis, you may need to follow an "adjusted" keto diet at first. The standard keto diet may not provide enough carbs to meet your needs. So, what's an "adjusted" keto diet?

An adjusted ketogenic diet is simply one where you adjust your macros to fit your needs before you're fat-adapted. (We will talk much more about _how many_ macros you need in the next chapter.)

Phase 1

Phase 1 of the keto workout strategy consists of eating an ample amount of healthy fats, some lean protein, and about one third or more of the day's allotted net carbs. (Again, we will talk about how to find your precise numbers in the next chapter.)

Phase 2

Phase 2 remains the same. Keto rebuilders (especially newbies) could benefit from eating 15-30 grams of fast-acting simple carbs 20-30 minutes before a workout (depending on the workout intensity). Some keto-adapted people will opt for MCT oil in place of these carbs, but it is highly dependent on the individual, how long they've been in ketosis, and how well they do without the simple carbs. Some people who fear being fatigued during a workout, eat berries beforehand.

Phase 3

After a workout, it's crucial to consume a good amount of protein (like whey) to help with protein synthesis. Some people also consume another one third or more of their daily max net carbs to assist muscles with glycogen recovery.

Chapter 4: Tools for the Fueling System

If the furnace in my house was not working, and I called an HVAC professional, I would expect them to come to my house with tools. Granted, tools aren't always "necessary," but they can certainly make the job go more smoothly and quickly. What's more, I would hope the professionals would bring the _correct_ tools—a pipe wrench, leak detector, digital thermometer, those types of things. It wouldn't be very beneficial if they came with hedge trimmers or a stump grinder.

It's the same when you're considering tools for the temple fueling system. They aren't "necessary" in most cases, but they can certainly make the rebuilding process go more smoothly and quickly. That is, if you have the _correct_ tools.

In this chapter, I will describe five products that I personslly think are the most state of the art "fuel tools" on the market today: Plexus Slim®, Plexus Block™, Plexus Balance™, Plexus Active™, and Plexus Edge®. **Again, it is recommended that you consult your doctor before taking <u>any</u> supplements to ensure they are safe for you. These are not approved by the FDA.**

Plexus Slim®

Plexus Slim® is known to many as the "pink drink." It comes in individual packets which you can open and pour directly into a bottle or glass of water. You then shake or stir vigorously for a delicious fruity-flavored drink. This pink, low-calorie drink should be consumed in the morning 30-60 minutes before breakfast. (Though it can also be taken later in the day before another meal if need be.) The ingredients in Plexus Slim® are known for their beneficial effects on glucose metabolism, as well as many other things. Let's go over a few of these key ingredients now.

Green Coffee Bean Extract

Green coffee bean extract (extracted from unroasted coffee beans) contains a substantial amount of chlorogenic acid, which is a naturally-occurring substance also found (to a lesser degree) in foods such as apples, plums, and cherries. Chlorogenic acid is not as prevalent in a roasted or ground coffee that you'd purchase in the supermarket, because the high heat involved in roasting the coffee beans breaks down much of the chlorogenic acid, thereby making it less available.

What makes chlorogenic acid beneficial as a "fuel tool" is that it can help decrease the absorption of sugar in the body. In fact, research shows it has a positive effect on blood sugar balance like some medications. For example, chlorogenic acid has been said to be an insulin sensitizer similar to metformin, with potency to stimulate the uptake of glucose molecules comparable to the antidiabetic drug rosiglitazone. (1)

The same research notes that high contents of chlorogenic acid can significantly reduce the risk for Type 2 Diabetes by 30%. It also reported that rats who were treated with chlorogenic acid had a decrease in cholesterol and triacylglycerol levels by 44% and 58%, and a decrease in liver triacylglycerols by 24%. In fact, in other studies, chlorogenic acid not only lowered cholesterol, but also significantly lowered body weight, visceral fat mass, plasma leptin, and insulin levels compared to the control group. (1)

Chromium Polynicotinate

Plexus Slim® also contains Chromium Polynicotinate. Chromium is referred to as an "essential trace mineral" because we need a small amount of it to maintain optimal health. One of the jobs of chromium is to help transport glucose into cells. Therefore, it plays a key role in balancing blood sugar and giving us steady energy. Chromium is not only needed to metabolize carbohydrates, but also protein and fat (including cholesterol). In fact, human studies show chromium supplementation can help lower levels of total cholesterol and low-density lipoprotein (LDL). (2)

It's been estimated by some, that up to 50% of the U.S. population is mildly deficient in chromium. I believe there are many possible reasons for this. First, the soil on many American crops is overused. Therefore, the soil itself often lacks nutrients like chromium. That means the produce grown in this deficient soil is often lacking nutrients also.

Additionally, several common medications such as H2 blockers, antacids, certain steroids, and proton-pump inhibitors can reduce chromium absorption or cause the body to flush it. What's more, wheat products are a major source of chromium, but there is a rising number of people developing wheat allergies and sensitivities who are adopting wheat-free diets, which can increase the risk of chromium deficiency.

Alpha Lipoic Acid

Plexus Slim® also contains an antioxidant called Alpha Lipoic Acid (ALA). ALA is present in every cell in the body. It is manufactured in small amounts in the mitochondria, where it is needed for a chain of reactions that create the ATP energy I mentioned at the beginning of this book. The problem is, the body produces less and less ALA as we age, and also when the immune system is weakened. So, the need for ALA increases in these instances.

In my opinion, ALA is one of the most underestimated antioxidants around. It does all your typical antioxidant type stuff (it searches out free radicals, fights inflammation, slows the aging process) but it also helps turn glucose into fuel. In fact, it is a proven tool for various blood sugar related issues, as studies have shown that ALA can help reduce fasting blood glucose (3), assist with diabetic neuropathy (4), and increase insulin sensitivity (5).

Keto and Slim

Clearly Plexus Slim contains many key ingredients that are known to help with glucose regulation. But that does not mean that Slim is *only* beneficial for those continuing to use glucose as fuel. It can also be beneficial for those transitioning into ketosis.

Just because you stop eating carbs doesn't mean blood sugar and insulin will just "go away." Glucose will still fluctuate while you are in ketosis. In fact, some people may notice that their fasting glucose levels rise in ketosis instead of fall.

This is because your muscles are typically the holding tank for stored glucose. When the body needs more fuel, it breaks down muscle to release this stored fuel. However, when you enter ketosis and start using fat for fuel (instead of glucose), your body "spares" the muscle. It doesn't break it down like it does when using glucose. It goes after fat stores instead. Therefore, after a while, the muscles stop taking in as much glucose because it's not needed. Because of this, the glucose from your veggies and other low carb foods is circulating in the blood, so is the glucose that the liver produces from protein via gluconeogenesis. This is why it's important to also look at insulin levels. The real "big picture" is glucose <u>and</u> insulin, not just glucose.

But I digress. My point is, glucose balance is still important in ketosis. This is especially true for people who are just starting the keto diet, who are pre-diabetic, or who have a history of erratic blood sugars, insulin resistance, or glucose intolerance. In these instances, Plexus Slim can be a beneficial tool to help you transition safely.

Garcinia Cambogia

Garcinia Cambogia is a bitter fruit from South Asia with high amounts of hydroxycitric acid (HCA). HCA blocks an enzyme that the body uses to make fat. This could prove beneficial for those in fat-burning ketosis. (Burning fat, but not making it, could equate to quicker weight loss.) HCA can also help raise serotonin, a neurotransmitter known to cause feelings of happiness and relaxation, as well as curb appetite and cravings.

Two Versions of Plexus Slim®

Plexus Slim® is available in two versions. There is the Plexus Slim® Microbiome Activating formula and the Plexus Slim® Hunger Control formula. Both have the same fuel-benefitting ingredients mentioned above, but each have different "extra" ingredients.

The Plexus Slim® Microbiome Activating formula also contains clinically studied xylooligosaccharides (XOS), which are prebiotic fibers that feed good microbes in the gut. I will talk extensively about the importance of gut microbes in the next phase.

The Plexus Slim® Hunger Control formula has polydextrose, which is a low-calorie soluble fiber that takes up space in the stomach and leaves slowly, helping you feel full longer. Some research suggests polydextrose may also have prebiotic potential, as well as contribute to increased energy and nutrient absorption, with positive effects on inflammatory bowel disease. (6) Also, studies have shown that polydextrose reduced bowel transit time (90%) and increased total weekly bowel frequency (from 3 times to 7 times a week) without inducing adverse gastrointestinal symptoms such as abdominal pain or bloating or induction of diarrhea. (6)

Plexus Block™

Plexus Block is a capsule packed full of ingredients that work to immediately block the absorption of up to 48% of the sugars and carbohydrates that you eat. This can be enormously beneficial for those of you who cannot adopt a ketogenic diet but who are trying to maintain stable glucose levels. It can also help those of you who are following a keto diet if you find yourself in a position where carbs are simply unavoidable (for example a work meeting, a wedding, etc.) Even if you consume carbohydrates and are kicked out of ketosis, there likely won't be as much glucose stored. Therefore, the transition back into ketosis could be quicker without as many keto flu symptoms.

Here's how Block™ works.

Plexus Block™ contains a proprietary brown seaweed blend, which helps reduce the glycemic index of carbs and sugars. If you remember from chapter two, the GI index illustrates how fast and how dramatically glucose is released (the rollercoaster versus a Sunday drive). Studies have shown that fasting blood glucose levels, and 2-hour blood glucose measurements were decreased significantly in those ingesting brown seaweed. (7)

Seaweeds are rich in dietary fibers, unsaturated fatty acids, and polyphenolic compounds. These bioactive compounds can inhibit various enzymes (like alpha-amylase and alpha-glucosidase) that turn carbs and sugars into glucose. (8)

Plexus Block™ also contains white kidney bean extract. Like brown seaweed, the white bean also produces an alpha-amylase inhibitor, which has been characterized and tested in numerous clinical studies. (9)

The beauty, though, is that while Plexus Block™ can block the absorption of some carbs and sugars, it does not block the absorption of nutrients. So, you get the best of both worlds.

In addition to these, Plexus Block™ also contains Chromium Picolinate which we've already discussed at length, as well as naturally occurring iodine that is in the seaweed. Iodine not only plays a role in maintaining insulin sensitivity (10), but animal studies have shown it can reduce glucose levels also. (11) What's more, iodine can be very beneficial for those with a low functioning thyroid, as thyroid cells take iodine, combine it with the amino acid tyrosine, and produce thyroid hormones T3 and T4.

Plexus Balance™

Similar to Plexus Block™, there is also Plexus Balance™. As the name suggests, Balance works to help *balance* blood sugar levels. It, too, can be taken before the largest meal of the day but works best when taken 20-30 minutes before the meal. Like Plexus Block™, Plexus Balance™ also contains White Kidney Bean Extract (Phaseolus vulgaris) which prevents the pancreas from secreting the enzyme amylase and helps manage the breakdown of carbohydrates and sugars.

Instead of chromium and brown seaweed, though, Balance has Common Bean Extract (Phaseolus vulgaris L.) that helps manage the breakdown of carbohydrates and sugars. It also has Cinnamon Bark Extract (Cinnamomum cassia) which also helps maintain healthy blood glucose levels. And it has Mulberry Leaf Extract (Morus alba L.) which helps to inhibit the breakdown of simple carbohydrates.

Each serving of Plexus Balance™ contains 1150 mg of this proprietary blend, compared to Block which has 500 mg of the seaweed blend, 200 mg of chromium, and 200 mg of white kidney bean extract per serving.

Both Plexus Block™ and Plexus Balance™ help to steady rollercoaster blood sugar levels but they accomplish this with different ingredients and concentrations. Plexus Block™ contains chromium as well as iodine (from seaweed) while Plexus Balance™contains a higher amounts of food extracts (cinnamon, cranberry, and mulberry). Those who cannot take chromium because of possible medication interaction might benefit more from Plexus Balance™. _Discuss these possibilities with your doctor before taking any supplements._

Tools for Increased Energy

As mentioned earlier, the purpose of any fuel system is to provide an efficient and stable source of energy. This is true when it comes to the temple of the body, also. That's why, if the temple fuel system is not working properly, it's not uncommon for some people to experience fatigue as a symptom of imbalanced blood sugar levels. The problem is it can take some time to rebuild the temple fuel system. So what can you do about fatigue in the meantime? How can you increase energy levels while in the process of rebuilding?

What Not to Do

For many people, the go-to remedy is "energy drinks." You know what they are. They are on the shelves of almost every grocery store, drug store, and gas station around. They are not hard to find. However, I personally do not choose these products for many reasons.

First and foremost, they are called "energy" drinks, but many contain around 27 grams of sugar per serving, and some contain two servings per can. That's 54 grams of sugar per can! Consuming that much sugar will inevitably cause rollercoaster blood sugar levels with dramatic peaks and falls. So, even though it is touted as an "energy" drink, it will likely result in increased fatigue later on. _(Note: many sugar free options also have sweeteners on my no-no list from earlier chapters.)_

Also, typical store-bought energy drinks usually contain a _synthetic_ form of caffeine. Yes, caffeine can be derived naturally from things such as coffee beans, tea leaves, and cacao beans. But, the form of caffeine traditionally used in energy drinks (and sodas, too) does not usually come from these sources. Rather, it is created in a lab.

The first synthetic caffeine lab was formed in 1945 by Monsanto (yes, the same company known for genetically modified crops). Other companies followed suit, but later all synthetic caffeine production moved abroad. Today, most synthetic caffeine is manufactured in overseas pharmaceutical plants in very "sketchy" conditions because foreign inspections are not usually required.

Also, synthetic caffeine powder undergoes several steps that are just not ideal, in my opinion. The process starts with urea, a compound that comes from ammonia. Then, it is exposed to several harsh chemicals during production. Finally, it is rinsed with things like sodium nitrite, acetic acid, sodium carbonate and chloroform. This last step is done because raw synthetic caffeine has a bluish glow which is not very appetizing.

Why is all this information important?

Because, even though synthetic and natural caffeine are almost indistinguishable at a molecular level, they are not identical in how they are created or digested. Natural caffeine grows in natural food sources and is still intact with its counterparts such as antioxidants, vitamins, and nutrients. Synthetic caffeine is absorbed in the digestive system much quicker than natural caffeine. So it gives a quicker boost, but also a quicker fall later on. It creates another digestive "rollercoaster," I guess you could say.

Too Much of a Not-So-Good Thing?

What's important to understand is that typical store-bought energy drinks often contain a *substantial* amount of this synthetic caffeine. Some brands have as much as 242 milligrams (mg) per serving—almost three times more caffeine than a cup of coffee, which only has about 85 mg. Many health organizations agree that up to 400 mg of caffeine a day is considered safe for most adults. So, on the surface, these energy drinks "seem" to be safe for consumption.

However, there is more to consider.

First, organizations agree 400 mg of caffeine **_a day_** is considered safe (100 mg a day for teens). That means, 400 mg of caffeine consumed over the course of many hours. The servings are typically spread out over a lengthy period of time—coffee at breakfast, iced tea at lunch, a mocha granola bar in the afternoon. But consuming 400 mg of caffeine in one energy drink (two servings in one can), takes place in a much shorter period of time and therefore has a much more dramatic effect on the body.

And remember synthetic caffeine in energy drinks digests faster than natural caffeine in coffee. So three times the amount of caffeine in a synthetic form, consumed all at once (not spread out over the day), is not just a bigger boost, but a faster boost. This is a lot harder on the body.

This is especially dangerous for children and teens, as one can of the typical energy drink could be **_four times_** more caffeine than the safe daily limit for teens. This could easily lead to caffeine toxicity, especially in people with a smaller build. Unfortunately, about 30% of U.S. teenagers (ages 12 through 17) still consume energy drinks on a regular basis anyway. (12)

What's also important to consider is that quick consumption also makes caffeine more addictive. You see, caffeine enhances dopamine signaling in the brain. Dopamine is a neurotramsmitter associated with feelings of pleasure and reward, as well as memory. So, when someone consumes caffeine, the brain experiences a flood of dopamine which not only produces feelings of pleasure and reward, but also records these feelings in memory. This causes a person to seek more caffeine, to experience those feelings of pleasure once again.

What's important to understand about addiction though, is the faster a substance or behavior takes place and elicits a reward, the more addictive it is. For example, cocaine that is injected is more addictive than cocaine that is snorted, because when injected it is assimilated into the body faster and provokes a quicker feeling of pleasure and reward.

In regards to caffeine, the same principle applies. An energy drink with 400 mg of synthetic caffeine that is consumed in 20 minutes is far more addictive than 400 mg of natural caffeine spread out over the course of 12 hours.

As with all addictions, the body develops a tolerance to the substance and must consume more of it to get the same reward. So, this explains why, after time, many people begin to "need" more than one energy drink a day. This becomes a huge problem because, while 400 mg of caffeine a day is considered safe for adults, some organizations say just 500 mg of caffeine is enough to cause caffeine toxicity in adults.

Other Reasons to Avoid Store-Bought Energy Drinks

The *amount* of synthetic caffeine is not the only reason to avoid store-bought energy products, in my opinion. Many of these energy drinks also contain other ingredients that increase the *effectiveness* of the synthetic caffeine. They also contain ingredients like guarana (from the seeds of a Brazilian shrub) that are stimulants similar to caffeine, but not classified as caffeine.

That means a label that claims to have just 200 mg of caffeine can be very deceiveing, because it often carries even more of a "punch" than it appears. This is especially important to remember for people who are already taking other stimulants, such as medications for Attention Deficit Disorder (ADD).

What's more, high consumption of caffeine also reduces insulin sensitivity, thereby increasing the risk of Type 2 Diabetes. Combine that with the high sugar content found in these drinks and the risks are even greater.

Caffeine can also influence hormone metabolism because sex hormones and caffeine are metabolized via similar enzymes. Some data suggests that caffeine can especially influence estrogen metabolism, as well as testosterone and sex hormone binding globlin (SHBG). (13) Therefore, high caffeine intake can potentially contribute to hormone imbalances in some people.

But again, it's not just the caffeine that is problematic, but the combination of multiple ingredients and the effects they have on each other. They can create a sort of 'perfect storm' in the body—and recent data confirms these risks.

One study published in the Journal of the American Heart Association found that caffeinated energy drinks altered the heart's electrical activity and raised blood pressure. (12) Another study done in Texas showed that after consuming just one energy drink, several participants experienced a decrease in blood vessel dialation—from 5.1 percent in diamaeter to 2.8 percent in diameter—which can reduce blood flow to various parts of the body, including the heart and brain. (14)

This can be especially dangerous before a workout if blood vessels in the heart do not dilate in order to allow enough blood to flow into the heart. Ironically (and unfortunately) some people consume energy drinks specifically for a pre-workout boost. Sometimes, parents even purchase these drinks for their kids before a sporting event.

Unknowingly people who consume these products are often doing far more harm to the body than good. In a prominent study over four years, the U.S. Substance Abuse and Mental Health Services Administration (SAMHSA) found a ten-fold increase in hospital-related emergency room visits due to energy drink consumption. People aged 18-24 had the highest number of ER visits, followed by those aged 26-39. (15)

Plexus Active™

Now that you know what **_not_** to do, let's go back to our original question: how can you (safely) increase your energy level while rebuilding your temple?

I personally have had great success using two Plexus "energy" tools in conjunction with the other Plexus "fuel" tools mentioned earlier. The first energy tool is Plexus Active™. This is a peach-mango flavored drink designed to increase alertness and wakefulness.

Okay, okay. Yes, I guess you could technically say it's an "energy drink" of sorts, but I prefer not to call it that because I do not want associate it with those other store-bought products. Active is too drastically different. Let me explain.

Plexus Active™ has only 25 calories, compared to the 200+ calories typically found in some energy drinks. Active does not have a high sugar content like typical energy drinks, either. In fact, Active has only 3 grams of sugar per serving because it is sweetened with honey powder, stevia, monk fruit extract, and a unique sweetener called trehalose. What makes these sweeteners better?

- Trehalose is naturally found in small amounts in mushrooms and honey. The source used in Active is derived from tapioca starch and is digested much slower than dextrose and sucrose.
- Monk fruit extract comes from the monk fruit like the name suggests. This is a small, round fruit grown in Southeast Asia that can provide a level of sweetness around 100–250 times greater than table sugar but with zero calories.
- Stevia, as I mentioned before, is a perennial herb native to South America with sweet-tasting leaves. It is standardized to 99% Rebaudioside A, then purified and crystallized into a compound typically 200 times sweeter than table sugar. It also has zero calories.

Also, Plexus Active contains 100 mg of _natural_ caffeine derived from green tea extract and yerba maté leaf extract. It has ActiGin, a compound of Panax notoginseng (ginseng) and Rosa roxburghii (chestnut rose) which, when combined with natural caffeine, help with endurance.*

Active also has L-Theanine, which is an amino acid most commonly found in green tea that helps to increase a sense of alertness and supports mental clarity and focus.* It has N-Acetyl L-Tyrosine, too, which provides an easily absorbed form of tyrosine. Tyrosine is an essential amino acid that is converted by the brain into neurotransmitters such as dopamine, adrenaline, and norepinephrine. Increasing these neurotransmitters is said to help improve memory and performance in stressful situations. (15)

In addition to that, Active also contains a mixture called S7. This is an antioxidant-rich blend of seven different plant extracts—green coffee bean extract, green tea extract, turmeric extract, tart cherry, blueberry, broccoli and kale.

What makes this significant is that S7 has been clinically shown to increase nitric oxide in the body by 175%. Our bodies already produce nitric oxide which acts as a vasodilator, signaling blood vessels to relax to increase blood flow. This helps the body's performance by delivering more oxygen, fuel, and other key nutrients to active muscles.

So, while energy drinks have been found to *decrease* blood vessel dialation and blood flow, Plexus Active helps to do the opposite—it helps *increase* dialation and blood flow. This makes Active a great option for pre-and post-workout support, whereas energy drinks are not a good option. In fact, Active also has citrulline, an amino acid the body makes when forming nitric oxide which is also involved in muscle recovery.

Active also contains a natural source of choline for brain power*, as well as many B vitamins, and vitamins A, C, and E.

Plexus Edge®

Another tool I occasionally use to increase energy is Plexus Edge®. Edge is a capsule with just three (very simple) key ingredients: L-Theanine, natural caffeine from coffea robusta, and Theacrine (as Patented TeaCrine®).

As mentioned, L-Theanine helps increase a sense of alertness and supports mental clarity. It also has a calming effect, making it an excellent choice to pair with natural caffeine, as it can help eliminate "jitters."*

Coffea robusta are coffee beans that have not been roasted. Therefore, not only does coffea robusta contain natural caffeine (just 90 mg in Plexus Edge), it also contains more chlorogenic acid. Chlorogenic acid can be helpful in balancing blood sugar levels, as noted in the section on Plexus Slim®.*

The third key ingredient in Plexus Edge® is theacrine, which naturally occurs in Kucha Tea leaves. Theacrine has been found to improve mood, decrease feelings of stress and irritability, and increase motivation, without disrupting sleep.*

Those are the only key ingredients in Plexus Edge® so you don't have to worry about interactions from a plethora of mysterious ingredients. Edge does not contain any artificial stimulants, dreadful sugars, sodium, or synthetic caffeine.

The Tool Shop

Perhaps now you are wondering how and where you can purchase these amazing tools. If you go to www.RebuildingYourTemple.com, click "Shop Plexus Now" or

"The Tool Shop," and you will be immediately directed to these and other temple tools. **OR, INSTEAD, GO TO THE WEBSITE OF THE PLEXUS AMBASSADOR WHO TOLD YOU ABOUT THIS BOOK.** This is very important. You will want a direct contact (who you know) who can guide you and help you problem-solve throughout the rebuilding process.

Regardless of what site you go to, you will notice there are three different ways you can purchase these and other temple tools.

1.) Buy Retail: This means you buy the products once at retail cost, and then you're done. There's no commitment to make another purchase. Honestly, I rarely recommend this to clients. Not only is it the most expensive way to buy, but most of the products are a 30-day supply, and it's rare that you will be able to completely rebuild your temple in 30 days. So, buying just once is like using tools for just half the job. It's like giving up your hammer and saw halfway through your home renovation. I don't recommend it.

2.) Buy as a Subscription: If you sign up for a subscription for these products, it means your products will auto-ship each month without you having to get online and make the purchase again. This strategy is cheaper than buying products at the retail price, and it is more convenient also. You won't have to worry about running out of products and being stuck without tools. What's more, you can cancel your future "auto-ship" orders at any time, and you will not be charged anything additional. There are no cancellation fees.

3.) Enroll as a Plexus Ambassador: As a health coach, this is probably what I recommend the most, for several reasons. One: when you become a Plexus ambassador, you can take advantage of wholesale pricing. Not only is this the cheapest way to buy, but you can potentially earn money back on your own purchases (which lowers your total cost even further). Two: you will be given your own Plexus website. You can use this to make your own purchases, or you can share this web site with friends and family to earn extra cash back through the Plexus referral program.

The Tool Manufacturer

Here is where many people go, *"Wait. Ambassador? Referral program? This sounds a lot like direct marketing, or MLM (muli-level marketing)."*

If you're thinking this, you're exactly right. It *is* direct marketing. It is MLM. But, please, don't close the book. Keep reading.

MLM has gotten a bad rap over the years, because a lot of companies have done it poorly and customers have gotten burned. If this is you, I'm sorry you had a bad experience like that, but please understand this is different. Not only is the Plexus compensation plan different from those other companies, but the company itself is different too. I can vouch for that, personally.

Listen, as a certified health coach and nutritionist, I WON'T offer just ANY products to my clients. This is my business, guys. My reputation. My passion. And my clients are my friends, my family, people I care about. I chose Plexus Worldwide as my product line after doing MUCH RESEARCH, because of several key reasons:

1.) I loved that Plexus was a health SYSTEM. The Plexus brand doesn't *just* offer protein, or *just* weight loss products, or *just* vitamins. I see Plexus as a whole-body health system, with products to address so many different things. As a health coach, this is of utmost importance to me because I have family members and clients with many different needs.

2.) I loved that the products are natural. Plexus ingredients are non-GMO, and the company doesn't use funky ingredients like corn syrup, sucralose, aspartame, carrageenan, etc. You'd be surprised how MANY health companies make products with cheap, harmful ingredients. They're everywhere! Those aren't things I will EVER recommend to my clients. Ever.

3.) I loved that Plexus products are tested! This is huge. HUGE. Plexus Worldwide has scientists on staff. There is research and testing to back products and ingredients. This way, when I recommend something to a client, I have DATA to back it up.

4.) I loved that Plexus is solid. If I'm going to partner with a company as a distributor, I want a solid company. I don't want to become a distributor of some fly-by-night brand that's going to disappear in a year. So you can imagine my relief when I found that, in 2013, Plexus had just experienced a 3-year growth rate of 16,458%, with a revenue of 159.8 million. This jumped to a revenue of 562 million in 2017, when they were recognized by Direct Selling News as #39 globally on its List of Top Revenue Generating Direct Selling Companies. *Inc. Magazine* also nominated Plexus Worldwide as one of the fastest growing private companies in America, ranking them number 8 on the list.

When I was searching for a "tool" brand, things like product span, ingredients, data, and company strength were important to me. When I discovered Plexus Worldwide, it was clear that this was the best option for my own personal health, the health of my family, and the health of my clients. Quite frankly, it was a no-brainer.

Now, let's get back to MLM. Perhaps you're still weary of the direct marketing industry, even though Plexus has proven to be a solid brand. Well, you should know that I actually chose Plexus Worldwide as my brand *because* they were a direct marketing company, not in spite of it. Allow me to explain.

If I offer a brand of "tools" that are just available via traditional means (you buy it retail when you need it with no option to enroll, get wholesale pricing, or earn cash back) then you will always have that supplement cost for the length of the rebuild. The problem with that is that some people won't be able to afford that extra cost. Others might be able to afford it for a little while, but then they'll have to forgo their tools halfway through the process when funds run out. Others may continue buying the tools they need, but then they'll have to cut costs on building materials to make room for these tools in their budget. (They'll have to resort to cheaper, processed food that is harmful to the body, and often works *against* the tools.) All of these situations will ultimately hinder the successful rebuilding of the temple.

Like a major home renovation project, resources are important. You can't complete a project you can't afford. The same is true when it comes to rebuilding your temple. That's why I *love* that these tools are available through a direct marketing channel. You have the ability to purchase your tools at the same wholesale price I do. (Imagine if you could go to Home Depot and buy the latest nail gun for the same price Home Depot bought it for!)

What's more, you can earn cash back on things you already buy at wholesale. It's like getting money back for buying the nail gun, and then using that money to buy more nails, a drill, and a saw… which in turn earns you even *more* cash back. It's also like telling your friends about your nail gun and getting even *more* cash back when they buy their tools.

These benefits are only possible through an MLM strategy. If you go to the local health store to purchase your temple tools, you will always have that set cost for as long as you rebuild (which is likely a marked-up cost, so that the distributor can profit). By enrolling with a direct marketing company, *you* become the distributor. You can purchase your tools from yourself and earn a profit. You can even potentially earn *more* cash back than you actually need for tools, and apply the excess towards quality building materials. Imagine how this could benefit your rebuild!

Getting Started

Maybe now you're convinced this is the way to go, but you're still unsure how to get started. How can you come up with the initial money you need to buy your first tool set and start rebuilding? It's a legitimate concern. Like I said, you can't build what you can't afford. Here are a few suggestions:

1.) Go through your expenses and look for areas where you can cut spending. Perhaps now you spend money daily on gourmet coffee, a morning breakfast sandwich, soda, tobacco, or energy drinks. Try to make your coffee and breakfast at home and please cut out the soda, tobacco and energy drinks. If you eat out for lunch each day, maybe you could start packing a lunch. If you spend a great deal of money at the salon, perhaps you could forgo the massage and do your nails and brows yourself this month. (Unfortunately, some people spend so much money painting the exterior of their temple, they have nothing left for the interior. But oftentimes, when the interior is taken care of first, the exterior gets a makeover too. I'll get more into this in later chapters.) The point is, prioritize. Look for unnecessary areas of spending that can be cut, at least for a time, so you can save enough to begin the rebuilding project. Your health is one of the most important things you will ever spend money on. All other expenses should pale in comparison.

2.) Get a group together from the start. Talk to your family and friends. See if there are three to five people who would want to "rebuild" with you. While the group support is enormously beneficial in terms of accountability and motivation, it can also prove financially beneficial. If you enroll as a Plexus ambassador, you can share your website with friends and family, and take advantage of the cash back incentives and/or the referral program. Talk to your ambassador about the details and how to go about this.

References:

(1) https://www.ncbi.nlm.nih.gov/pmc/articles/PMC3766985/
(2) https://www.ncbi.nlm.nih.gov/pmc/articles/PMC1002252/
(3) https://www.ncbi.nlm.nih.gov/pubmed/21666939
(4) https://www.ncbi.nlm.nih.gov/pubmed/23678828
(5) https://www.ncbi.nlm.nih.gov/pubmed/15913551
(6) https://www.ncbi.nlm.nih.gov/pmc/articles/PMC5037538/
(7) https://www.ncbi.nlm.nih.gov/pmc/articles/PMC2815322/
(8) https://www.ncbi.nlm.nih.gov/pmc/articles/PMC4557030/
(9) https://www.ncbi.nlm.nih.gov/pmc/articles/PMC3071778/

(10) Küpper, Frithjof & Schweigert, Nina & Ar Gall, E & Legendre, J.-M & Vilter, Hans & Kloareg, B. (1998). Iodine uptake in Laminariales involves extracellular, haloperoxidase-mediated oxidation of iodide. Planta. 207. 163-171. 10.1007/s004250050469.

(11) Rajendran D, Pattanaik AK, Khan SA, et al. Iodine Supplementation of Leucaena leucocephala Diet for Goats. II. Effects on Blood Metabolites and Thyroid Hormones. Asian-Australas J Anim Sci. 2001;14(6):791-6

(12) https://www.ahajournals.org/doi/full/10.1161/JAHA.118.011318

(13) https://onlinelibrary.wiley.com/doi/pdf/10.1002/cncr.24328https://www.sciencedaily.com/releases/2018/11/181105081738.htm

(14) http://www.advanceer.com/link-energy-drinks-er-visits

(15) https://www.healthline.com/nutrition/tyrosine#section1

Phase 2:

Rebuilding the Electrical System

Materials: Saturated Fats, Monounsaturated Fats, Polyunsaturated Fats (Omega 6s and Omega 3s), Organic Fruits, and Organic Vegetables

Tools: Plexus MegaX, Plexus Ease, Plexus xFactor Plus, Plexus Nerve

Chapter 5: The Importance of Healthy Fats

Congratulations! You made it through Phase One of the rebuild! I hope you were able to pull out some pertinent information that you can share with your doctor and begin to implement. It's now time to move on to Phase Two. Let's get working on the wiring!

In a typical house, the electrical system is comprised of wires and a panel. In the temple of the body, the electrical system consists of the nervous system and the "panel" of the brain. While awake, the brain generates between 10 and 23 watts of power (1) or enough energy to power a light bulb. Believe it or not, we are electrical! Everything in the body is connected through nerve cells, chemical messengers, and electrical impulses. You could say that the nervous system "wires" us together.

Some of you, who are mostly interested in "rebuilding" for weight loss, might be tempted to just skip by this phase assuming it is irrelevant for your goals. Please don't do that. This is an important system when it comes to weight loss, too.

You see, the brain can send messages to fat tissue via nerve cells in the sympathetic nervous system. These fat cells produce the hunger hormone leptin, which travels up to the brain to lower appetite and boost metabolism. The brain then sends signals back down to the fat cells when it's time to break down fats into energy.

In fact, a recent study in mice showed that stimulating these nerves stimulated fat breakdown. (2) It mimicked the effect of increasing leptin in the mice. So, a healthy nervous system and a healthy brain are very important when it comes to a complete weight loss strategy, as well as overall health—and isn't that *really* the goal?

So, now the question is: how do we rebuild the wiring of the temple? How do we take care of the brain and nervous system to ensure they stay healthy and working properly?

First, we have to "feed" the brain and nervous system. We do that by consuming _healthy_ fats. This topic is crucial for those of you adopting a ketogenic diet because up to 80% of your calories could be coming from fat. But it is also important for those of you who are still running on glucose too. Fat is not only an excellent fuel source for the body; it is also vital for the brain and nervous system. While the brain itself is 70% water (it is susceptible to dehydration, which we'll talk about in later chapters) about 60% of the "dry" weight of the brain is made up of fat.

This, in my opinion, is the great tragedy that has resulted from the "fat fear" of the last few decades. Because supposed health "experts" have been vilifying fat and championing a low-fat diet, people have been avoiding ALL fat, even healthy fat. By doing so, many people have been inadvertently depriving their brain and nervous system of a much-needed macronutrient.

The fact is, healthy fats insulate the axons of neurons, which transmit brain signals. This insulation is called myelin sheath, which protects your nerves. Think of it like the insulation surrounding an electrical wire. 80% of this is made up of fat from our diet! If this "insulation," or myelin, becomes damaged, it can result in diseases such as MS and Guillain-Barre syndrome.

Plugging In

Another thing to keep in mind is that brain cells communicate via a sender/receiver network. Cell membranes have receptor sites designed and shaped for specific fat molecules. Think of a cell as one of those round "shape sorters" that toddlers often play with. The toy comes with shaped blocks that fit perfectly into the shaped holes. Well, a natural fatty acid will fit nicely into a cell receptor just like a shaped block will fit nicely into the same shaped hole.

Different cells have different types of receptors, though—like different sorters might have different shaped holes. Each receptor has different functions too. Regardless, once the fatty acid "plugs" into the receptor, that's when the "magic" happens. (It's like when a plug enters an outlet.)

For example, when a long-chain fatty acid "plugs" into a receptor known as GPR40, it can stimulate insulin secretion from pancreatic cells as well as neurons in the cerebral cortex, hippocampus, amygdala, hypothalamus, cerebellum and spinal cord. (3)

GPR120, on the other hand, is a receptor that stimulates secretion from colon and immune cells; GPR119 and GPR84 are nutritional receptors, and GPR43 promotes energy and suppresses fat accumulation. As you can see, it's important to healthy fats, so that fatty acids can plug in and stimulate "action" in the body.

Unfortunately, though, not all fats fit into receptors—take, for example, man-made fats. To increase the shelf life of food, manufacturers will take a liquid, unsaturated fat (like vegetable oil) and add a hydrogen atom to it. This transforms it into a saturated fat that is more solid (like margarine or shortening).

But during this hydrogenation process, the hydrogen atoms are "transported" across the fat molecule to a new location, making it an oddly-shaped saturated fat called "trans fat." Dr. Udo Erasmus describes a trans-fat as a "molecule that has its 'head on backward'" in his book *Fats that Heal, Fats that Kill.*

The problem is: these now oddly-shaped hydrogenated fatty acids will still try to enter receptor sites. It's like forcing an oval block into a circle hole, or a three-pronged plug into a two-pronged outlet. This will either damage the cell or clog the receptor so that healthy fats cannot plug into the cell membrane with much-needed nutrients.

If the cell becomes damaged enough, even healthy fatty acids will no longer fit. And without enough good fatty acids, the cell membrane can become weak, which can lead to many various degenerative diseases.

Unfortunately, hydrogenated fats are not the only misshaped and problematic fats. There are now what's called interesterified fats. These are made by combining natural vegetable oil with stearic acid (a saturated fatty acid typically from animals) to make it more like a hardened fat with a longer shelf life. Once again, this changes the molecular structure of the oil. The end product then does not resemble anything found in nature and does not fit receptors.

While these new fats are touted as being "free of trans fat," they still contain harmful residues that cause cell damage and raise cholesterol. Additionally, studies show that these interesterified fats even raise blood glucose and reduce insulin production. (4)

The Saturated Fat Villain

Next, you are probably expecting me to list saturated fat in my litany of "bad fats." Saturated fat is one of the most vilified fats by the media and most shunned fats by consumers. But it is NOT on my "bad" list. In fact, saturated fat is on my "good" list. I know, I know. This is likely surprising to you. But let me explain.

Saturated fats are natural fats found in nature...just like monounsaturated fats and polyunsaturated fats, which I will talk about next. Saturated fats are found in foods such as eggs, butter, dark chocolate, and coconut oil, to name a few. Natural saturated fats are not altered; they don't have their "head on backward." They were given to us (for us), by the architect of our temples. Therefore, unlike misshapen trans fats and interesterified fats, the body knows exactly what to do with saturated fats. In fact, the body welcomes them and needs them for many important jobs, especially when it comes to the brain and nervous system.

You don't have to take my word for it, though. There are plenty of medical experts that have already published a wealth of information to support this.

The Brain

According to bariatric Drs. Michael and Mary Dan Eades (as cited on the blog of New York Times and Wall Street Journal bestselling author, Tim Ferriss), "...the lion's share of the fatty acids in the brain are actually saturated. A diet that skimps on healthy saturated fats robs your brain of the raw materials it needs to function optimally." (5)

They also add, "Certain saturated fats, particularly those found in butter, lard, coconut oil, and palm oil, function directly as signaling messengers that influence the metabolism, including such critical jobs as the appropriate release of insulin. And just any old fat won't do. Without the correct signals to tell the organs and glands what to do, the job doesn't get done or gets done improperly." (5)

Heart Disease and High Cholesterol

Drs. Michael and Mary Eades are a husband and wife duo who have authored 14 books in the fields of health, nutrition, and exercise and who have founded a chain of ambulatory out-patient family care clinics called Medi-Stat Medical Clinics. And, they make a convincing push for healthy, brain-friendly saturated fats.

Perhaps, this still doesn't set your mind at ease, though. Maybe you're still wondering, "What about heart disease and high cholesterol?"

This seems to be the biggest and most common fear associated with saturated fat consumption. And while I realize this is a chapter on the brain and nervous system (I don't want to get too far off that topic), I would be remiss if I did not touch on other saturated fat benefits as well.

According to the Eades duo, adding healthy saturated fats to the diet reduces lipoprotein (a) or Lp(a), which correlates strongly with risk for heart disease. "Currently there are no medications to lower this substance," they say, "and the only dietary means of lowering Lp(a) is eating saturated fat. Bet you didn't hear that on the nightly news. Moreover, eating saturated (and other) fats also raises the level of HDL, the so-called good cholesterol." (5)

This is important because HDL (good) cholesterol removes LDL (bad) cholesterol from the arteries. It works like a cholesterol cleanup crew, carrying LDL back to the liver where it is broken down or passed out of the body as waste. So if eating more saturated fat means gaining more HDL cholesterol, as the Eades couple say, than that means more cleanup of arteries.

Dr. Mark Hyman, also stated, "Saturated fat is not linked to heart disease in the absence of refined (starchy) carbs and sugar, and in the presence of omega 3 fats. And review after review after independent review of the research shows that there seems to be no link between saturated fats and heart disease. In fact, a recent large review of the research found that the higher the saturated fat intake, the lower the risk of stroke." (6)

The Liver

It's been widely accepted that saturated fat consumption can be problematic for the liver, especially for those who have fatty liver disease. However, Dr. Hyman had this to say: "To prevent or reverse fatty liver, you'll want to cut processed carbs and increase healthy fat intake, especially saturated – yes, saturated – fats from healthy foods like coconut and grass-fed beef." (7)

Drs. Michael and Mary Dan explain why. "Adding saturated fat to the diet has been shown in medical research to encourage the liver cells to dump their fat content...Additionally, saturated fat has been shown to protect the liver from the toxic insults of alcohol and medications...Polyunsaturated vegetable fats do not offer this protection." (5)

The Lungs

According to internationally renowned lipid chemistry expert Mary G. Enig, Ph.D., FACN, CNS, healthy saturated fat can also benefit the lungs. According to Enig, the human lung surfactant (coating) is made up of fat—100 percent of which is saturated fatty acids. "When people consume a lot of partially hydrogenated fats and oils," she says, "the trans fatty acids are put...where the body normally wants to have saturated fatty acids and the lungs may not work effectively. Some research has suggested that trans fatty acids are causing asthma in children." (8)

The Immune System and Nutrients

It has been found that healthy saturated fats are also helpful for the immune system. Drs. Michael and Mary Eades explain, "Saturated fats found in butter and coconut oil (myristic acid and lauric acid) play key roles in immune health. Loss of sufficient saturated fatty acids in the white blood cells hampers their ability to recognize and destroy foreign invaders, such as viruses, bacteria, and fungi." (5)

What's more, it's important to remember that many vitamins (like vitamin K, A, D, and E) are fat-soluble vitamins. That means they don't dissolve in water (like water-soluble vitamins) but are absorbed with higher-fat foods, and then stored in fatty tissue and the liver. Not eating enough fat, therefore, can inhibit the absorption of these crucial vitamins when supplementing. Natural sources of fat-soluble vitamins, though, already come with the necessary fat for absorption. For example, vitamin A is present in animal liver and butter; vitamin D3 is present in animal fats; vitamin E is present in almonds and hazelnuts; vitamin k is present in liver and egg yolks.

The Prosecutor

For some of you, the information contained in this chapter is turning everything you thought you knew upside down. You may have thought that lower-fat margarine was the healthier option, not realizing it was a misshapen trans-fat potentially harmful to your lungs. You may have even thought that butter was the devil, not realizing it provides fat-soluble vitamins (10% of the Daily Value of vitamin A) and boosts the immune system. If you thought this way, know you are not alone. Saturated fat has been widely misunderstood by many Americans for many years. But why? With all these benefits how on earth did saturated fat ever become a villain in the first place?

It started back in the 1950s when physiologist Ancel Keys, Ph. D published a paper linking saturated fat with increasing rates of heart disease and death. The problem with his writing was that he studied 22 countries, but he only used data from six of them. If he would have included the data from the other 16 countries the study would have clearly shown that healthy fat consumption reduces the number of deaths from coronary heart disease, not increases it. In fact, the complete data would have also shown that those who consumed the highest percentage of saturated fat had the lowest risk of heart disease. (9) (10)

With that paper, Ancel Keys put saturated fat on trial with misinformation and the jury of the American people bought it hook, line, and sinker. The media jumped on board, and the erroneous information began its wide-spread circulation. Health professionals and consumers then latched on too, and food companies began making lower-fat (trans-fat) alternatives.

The gauntlet was thrown down, and saturated fat was officially condemned by the general public.

The good news is science prevails. Decades of ongoing research has since vilified the trans-fat alternative, and so people are starting to rethink things. More and more studies are being conducted, and the word is getting out: saturated fat was falsely accused.

For example, 21 studies followed a total of 347,747 participants for 5-23 years and found no significant evidence that dietary saturated fat is associated with an increased risk of heart disease or cardiovascular disease. (6) Another Japanese study followed 58,453 Japanese adults for 14 years and found the same thing: the intake of saturated fat was not associated with an increased risk of heart disease. However, the study did reveal that those who ate more saturated fat had a lower risk of stroke. (11) These more recent studies are echoing what Keys' paper should have said, had he included all the data.

Those Who Should Proceed with Caution

I've said it before, and I'll say it again: what works for one person may not work for everyone. The same is true here, too, as it relates to saturated fat. While saturated fat has many health benefits, there are some who might need to proceed with caution. So, again, it is crucial to discuss everything with your doctor before changing your diet.

As I mentioned earlier in this book, some people have a genetic makeup that makes digesting saturated fat difficult. Take the APoE gene, for example. The APoE gene determines how the body metabolizes cholesterol—either quickly, efficiently, or slowly. Think of it like an Uber that shuttles cholesterol. Some Uber APoE genes are quick drivers; some are efficient; some are slow.

There are three different variations of the APoE gene (APoE2, APoE3, and APoE4). The APoE2 variant is like an Uber in a racecar. It instructs the body to shuttle cholesterol very quickly. Therefore, people with APoE2 typically have low cholesterol and do well on high-fat diets in the absence of refined carbs and sugar.

The APoE3 variant is considered normal. It's like an Uber in a new mid-size sedan. It instructs the body to shuttle cholesterol efficiently, just as it should. It gets the job done, not too fast and not too slow. Therefore, people with APoE 3 typically do well eating healthy fat also, while still maintaining proper cholesterol levels.

Then there is the APoE4 variation. APoE4 is like the Uber that shows up in a lemon that can't accelerate over 30 MPH. APoE4 instructs the body to metabolize or shuttle cholesterol very slowly. Therefore, people with the APoE4 variation have a greater risk of high cholesterol build-up, and consequently, a greater risk of cardiovascular issues, even a reduced response to statins. So, these people can have a difficult time with saturated fat consumption and might do better eating more monounsaturated and polyunsaturated fat, instead of saturated fat (which I will discuss later in this chapter).

Also, because APoE is the primary cholesterol carrier in the brain, having ApoE4 poses a higher risk of Alzheimer's disease because of resulting brain inflammation and oxidative stress from cholesterol buildup.

Now, it's important to note that we inherit one of these APoE genes from each parent. Therefore, we each have two copies...one of six possible combinations. Some people have two copies of APoE2 or two copies of APoE3. Others have an E2/E3 combo or E3/E4 combo, and so forth and so on.

Why does this combination matter? Because it affects the risk factor. Someone with a combo of a fast E2 and a slow E4 is at a higher risk than someone with two copies of a fast E2. And someone with two copies of a slow E4 poses the most significant risk of all the possible combinations.

If you're concerned about your genetic risk because of a personal or family history of heart disease, stroke, or high cholesterol, talk to your doctor about genetic testing. You can also order genetic testing online yourself from places like 23andme.com.

I personally have done genetic testing (online) for myself and my family, and the knowledge it provides is invaluable when it comes to formulating an individualized diet/health plan. As I said, we are all unique individuals and what works for one person may not work for another. I have seen this in my own family, with my children, even though they all come from the same gene pool. Knowledge is power, guys. So, I will talk more about genetic testing later on.

The Omega See Saw

The body can produce many different kinds of natural fatty acids, but there are certain ones that you _need_ to get from your diet because your body is not able to make them on its own. These are called essential fatty acids (because it is "essential" that we eat them since we cannot make them.)

The two essential fatty acids are linoleic acids (known as omega-6 fatty acids) and alpha-linolenic acids (known as omega-3 fatty acids). These both come from polyunsaturated fats. For optimal health, these omega 6s and omega 3s should be balanced 1:1 in the diet. For every omega 6 you eat, you should have an omega 3 to balance it.

Most Americans don't have a problem getting enough omega 6 fatty acids because they are found in common foods such as vegetable oils, peanut oil, various seeds, meat, and dairy. This is good because omega 6 fatty acids can help lower "bad" (LDL) cholesterol levels, raise "good" (HDL) cholesterol levels, and reduce the risk of cancer and heart disease.

Unfortunately, omega 3s are not eaten as often because they are found in more uncommon things like salmon, cod, chia seeds, and flaxseed. Because these are not eaten as often, the 1:1 ratio can be skewed, sometimes as dramatically as 20:1, even 50:1, in favor of omega 6s.

This becomes a problem because the outside layer of a cell is made up mostly of omega 3s, which have several essential functions. These omega 3s can stimulate the GPR120 receptor, which reduces inflammation in immune cells and enhances insulin sensitivity. Omega 3s can "turn on" genes for fat burning and "turn off" genes for fat storing. They support thyroid function and are used to make hormones like testosterone and estrogen. In fact, fat, in general, is involved in the gene signaling responsible for hormone balance.

Omega 3s are also crucial for eye health, reducing triglycerides, blood pressure, and the buildup of plaque in the arteries. They help reduce joint pain, fight depression and ADHD, boost immunity and mood, improve skin, balance blood sugar levels, and reduce the risk of Alzheimer's.

While both types of polyunsaturated fats are important, what is perhaps even more important is the 1:1 balance. Research has shown that an out-of-balance omega see-saw (high in omega 6 fatty acids, low in omega 3s) can encourage chronic inflammation and increase the risk of asthma, allergies, diabetes, and arthritis. It can alter immunity and gene expression. (12) And it is believed this imbalance in omegas can contribute to autoimmunity, neurodegenerative diseases, depression, learning disorders, attention and hyperactivity issues, even violence.

So, please understand that the number of fats you calculated in chapter 3 is way more than just a number. It's not enough to eat a certain _amount_ of fat. You have to eat a certain _kind_ of fat: polyunsaturated, _essential_ fatty acids. And you have to eat them in the right proportion.

Therefore, you have to go a step further when it comes to macro tracking.

If you are sticking to your fat macros (and getting your 45 grams each day), but these fats are coming from trans-fats and interesterified fats… then yes, you might be providing your temple with the right _amount_ of energy, but not the right _kind_. You might inadvertently be wreaking havoc on your wiring system.

I know, this might sound like this is getting very complicated, but once you know what to look for, choosing healthy fats will become second nature to you. I promise. That's why I encourage you to get the *Rebuilding Your Temple Workbook* so you can take notes as you go, so you can study this information, and take it shopping with you.

If you're feeling overwhelmed, let me summarize thus far:

- Avoid hydrogenated fats, trans fats, and interesterified fats like the plague.
- Look carefully at the polyunsaturated (essential fatty acids) you consume. Aim for a 1:1 omega 6 to omega 3 balance.

For most of you, it will not be difficult to get in enough omega 6s. But you will probably need to work harder to get enough omega 3s. It is recommended that we consume a fist-sized portion of seafood at least three times a week. But if that is not doable, below is a chart of some other options.

Food	Approx Omega 3s	Serving
Atlantic Mackerel	6,500 mg	1 cup cooked
Salmon Fish Oil	4,400 mg	1 tablespoon
Cod Liver Oil	2,300 mg	1 tablespoon
Walnuts	2,200 mg	¼ cup
Chia seeds	2,100 mg	1 tablespoon
Herring	1,600 mg	3 ounces
Alaskan Salmon	1,500 mg	3 ounces
Flax Seeds	1,300 mg	1 tablespoon
Albacore Tuna	1,200 mg	1 tablespoon
White Fish	1,100 mg	3 ounces
Sardines	1,100 mg	3.75 ounces
Hemp Seeds	800 mg	1 tablespoon
Anchovies	700 mg	2 ounces
Natto	600 mg	½ cup
Egg Yolks	100 mg	½ cup

How to Buy Seafood

As you can see from the chart above, various types of fish are often highest in omega 3 fatty acids. Perhaps you are wondering: what makes seafood so high in these? Well, as the adage goes, "you are what you eat." This is true for fish, too.

Cold-water fish eat algae (which is rich in omega 3 fatty acids), and so they end up with high amounts of omega 3s in their tissue. Likewise, salmon eat pink crustaceans called krill, also rich in omega 3 fatty acids, and so they end up with omega 3s in their tissue too. When we consume these omega-rich fish, then, these omegas transfer to us.

To make it even better, algae and krill are rich in a specific kind of omega 3s—EPA (eicosapentaenoic acid) and DHA (docosahexaenoic acid). Of the 11 different types of omega 3 fatty acids out there, these are by far the two most important ones. EPA and DHA are the building blocks of cell membranes and are responsible for the majority of the benefits I mentioned earlier in this chapter. So, this provides a direct benefit for us when we consume the fish that have eaten these omegas.

Now, before you rush out seafood shopping, there is something you should know: not all cold-water fish eat algae and not all salmon eat krill. Farm-raised fish typically do not eat either of these or at least very little of it. More often than not, they eat genetically modified grains and legumes. So, instead of omega 3s, these farm-raised fish are eating high amounts of herbicides. And quite frankly, so are you when you consume them. (Additionally, farm-raised salmon that do not eat pink krill, do not have the same pink color that wild salmon do, so they are often injected with a synthetic pigment too. Yummy.)

Because of this, farm-raised seafood does not have the same nutrient value as wild-caught seafood. In fact, it has been found that farm-raised salmon has up to 50% less omega 3s than wild-caught salmon. Before you say, "well, it's better than nothing," let me explain the other problems with farm-raised seafood.

Farmed fish are raised in pens, in large quantities. They are packed together with very little space, unlike wild-caught fish that grow unimpeded in their natural habitat. This "pen environment" creates an easy breeding ground for bacteria and diseases like Sea Lice. To prevent this, the farm fish are often given antibiotics, chemicals, and more pesticides—which, yes, are often transferred to us when we eat them.

Remember: you are what you eat. Various chemicals found in farmed seafood can interfere with immune response, cause inflammation, disrupt hormones, and contribute to metabolic disorders.

So, how do you choose healthy seafood? First and foremost, DO NOT buy farm-raised anything. That's my personal and professional opinion. Look for "wild-caught" on the label. But you should also know that the term "wild" has been misused and so you will also want to look for a logo from the Marine Stewardship Council verifying that it actually is wild-caught like the label claims.

If you are trying to buy salmon and it does not say farm or wild, and it does not have a logo, choose Alaskan salmon. Alaska takes the quality of their seafood very seriously, and their salmon is not allowed to be farmed (not even canned Alaskan salmon is allowed to be farmed). Sockeye salmon cannot be farmed either, so these are two keywords to look for when shopping (though sockeye is unmistakable regardless of the label because it has a very bright pinkish-red color which is very different from other types of peach-colored salmon.)

This is also something to keep in mind when eating out at restaurants since it has been estimated that 90-95% of salmon at restaurants is farmed, even when labeled "wild." Look for Alaskan or Sockeye on the menu or ask your server for more information.

If you are still unsure, you can go to www.seafoodwatch.org and research a brand or an establishment to determine if it is a quality form of seafood. They even have an app you can download on your phone.

Reading Labels

In most cases, all three types of fatty acids (saturated, monounsaturated, and polyunsaturated) are present in fatty food, at the same time. Like a multi-stringed necklace, these fatty acid chains are attached to a bar-like structure, called a glycerol molecule. This is where you get the term triglycerides. "Tri" means three fatty acids; and "glycerides" means on one glycerol molecule.

They are classified differently, though, based on their makeup. Whichever fatty acid is most abundant determines its name. Take olive oil, for example. It's a triglyceride, meaning it has all three fatty acids. But it's comprised of approximately 72% monounsaturated, 12% polyunsaturated, and 16% saturated fatty acids. Therefore, it's classified as a monounsaturated fat because that is what is most abundant.

Now, there are also what's called diglycerides and monoglycerides. As the name implies, these fats have only one or two chains of fatty acids, instead of three. These start as a triglyceride that is then synthesized via catalytic transesterification—a big word that basically means it is processed. The result is an oil byproduct that contains, yep, you guessed it: _trans fat_.

The problem is these mono and diglycerides are used as emulsifiers (ingredients that help water and oil bind together better in recipes). Because of this, they do not fall under "trans fat" labeling requirements, because they aren't classified as fats. They're classified as emulsifiers.

Also, companies are allowed to list trans fats as "0" if the foods contain less than 0.5 grams of trans fat per serving. So, many packaged foods that list "0" trans fats on their nutrition labels actually do contain these artificial fats. (Some even list trans-fatty acids or mono- and diglycerides right there in fine print in the ingredients list.)

The problem is two-fold. One, to make the numbers equal less than .5 grams, they typically make the serving size unreasonably small. So, you end up eating far more than .5 grams because you eat far more than what they consider to be one serving. Two, if many food manufacturers are doing this, and you're eating several different processed foods each day, then accumulatively you're not just eating "small amounts" of trans fat anymore.

The same is true for interesterified fats. Companies do not need to list it on the label. Instead, they might use terms like "high stearate" or "stearic rich fats" in the ingredients list, which are code words for interesterified fat. What's even worse, some oils like palm oil, palm kernel oil, vegetable oil, and fully hydrogenated vegetable oil do not even need to list code names. They can be listed as is and still potentially contain interesterified or trans fat.

This is another reason why it's important to pay very close attention to what kind of fat you are consuming. Not only do you have to look at the grams of fat in the nutrition label—and whether it's polyunsaturated, saturated, monounsaturated or trans—but you also have to look at the ingredients list below it. You need to read every ingredient like a detective.

If you see vegetable, palm, soybean, or canola listed, chances are it could have trans or interesterified fat. If you see anything with the below words, it almost certainly does. Put it back on the shelves.

- Diglycerides
- Monoglycerides
- Hydrogenated
- Partially hydrogenated
- Stearate
- Stearic
- Trans

Shopping for Omega Supplements

By now, some of you may be feeling discouraged thinking about how many omega 3s you need to consume to balance out your omega 6 consumption. It may feel daunting to you, especially if you are a vegetarian or vegan, if you have an allergy, or if you just can't stand the taste of seafood. These are two instances where it's probably not possible to increase your weekly seafood intake. I get that.

But, that doesn't change the importance of omega 3s, which remember, are "essential" because your body cannot make them on its own. In fact, according to a study done by Harvard University, an omega-3 fatty acid deficiency is one of the top 10 preventable causes of death in America, resulting in up to 96,000 deaths each year. (13) So, if you don't eat seafood or seeds, we need to talk about supplements.

There are MANY omega 3 supplements (many rebuilding tools) on the market nowadays—but not all are created equal. So it is crucial to go over it all. First, let's look at omega 3 fatty acids again. As I said, the two most important types of omega 3s are EPA and DHA. These are both long-chain fatty acids.

There is also what's known as Alpha-linolenic Acid (ALA), which is a plant-based omega 3 (found in seeds, leafy vegetables, and walnuts). This is an omega 3, yes, but it is a _short_-chain fatty acid. This means your body has to add carbons to it to convert it into the longer-chained EPA and DHA that are so essential. And quite frankly, this process is very inefficient. Some studies suggest only 8% of ALA is converted to EPA, and 0-4% is actually converted to DHA. (14)

To make it even trickier, healthy saturated fats are needed to make the conversion from ALA to EPA and DHA. So, eating foods like coconut can help the conversion rate, but it's still not very efficient. The percentage may also be slightly higher for women than men. But still, we can't deny the importance of getting essential EPA and DHA from food.

But! Before you run out to the local drug store and purchase the cheapest omega 3 product on the shelf, we need to talk about the differences between omega supplements... because there ARE differences.

The most popular go-to for omega 3 supplementation is fish oil. However, just like there are significant differences between farmed fish and wild-caught fish, there are also differences between various fish oil supplements.

Like any oil, fish oil can become rancid. This is easy to identify by the strong, fishy taste and smell. Fresh fish oil should be mild smelling/tasting. It should contain vitamin E (an antioxidant to keep it fresh), and it should be refrigerated in a glass bottle to prevent oxidation. It should also list a breakdown of both EPA and DHA, not just the total omega 3 amount.

This is extremely important. Rancid fish oil is very hazardous to your health at the cellular level. It can also increase your risk of heart disease, atherosclerosis, and blood clots. Unfortunately, though, there is a lot of rancid fish sold on store shelves these days. If you take a fish oil supplement currently, I recommend checking the brand through a third-party company. I personally have used ConsumerLab.com to obtain this information. I paid approximately $20 for the full report, and it was well worth the cost.

For Vegetarians

If you are vegetarian and do not want to take a fish oil supplements, you can opt for a plant-based omega 3 product. Algal oil, for example, comes from algae and has very high concentrations of DHA, which is especially good for the brain. Krill oil, while it is often more expensive, is high in both EPA and DHA omega 3 fatty acids. In fact, krill oil is almost identical to fish oil in that respect, except it is more bioavailable (more absorbable), and also has more antioxidants than fish oil.

What's more, astaxanthin (the antioxidant in krill oil) is said to be 6,000 times higher than vitamin C and 550 times higher in vitamin E. (15) The one downfall is that it does not have the vitamin D content that fish oil typically has.

Another option would be the Plexus omega product. Plexus makes a vegetarian omega called MegaX™ that contains AHIFLOWER® Oil which contains omega-3 Stearidonic Acids (SDAs). SDAs have been shown to convert to long-chain omega 3 fatty acids more efficiently than flaxseed ALA because SDAs bypass a conversion step involving a liver enzyme.

If you are a vegetarian considering an omega and have pain associated with inflammation, you might also consider Plexus Ease® in addition to the MegaX. Ease contains green-lipped mussel. Green-lipped mussel typically contains long-chain DHAs and EPAs, as well as rare, 19-carbon furan fatty acids that act as powerful antioxidants. Together, these block the production of the immune chemicals (leukotrienes) that trigger inflammation, and they block key enzymes similar to the way aspirin and NSAIDs do. (16) So, this can be beneficial in terms of a natural pain reliever. (I've used it myself many times with great success.) I will talk more about Plexus Ease® in the next chapter.

As always, before you supplement with omega-3 fatty acids of any kind, make sure you consult your doctor, especially if you are taking medications, to prevent any possible interactions.

The Electrical Fire

Another thing to take into consideration when it comes to unhealthy fats is inflammation. It's no secret that trans fats and interesterified fats contribute to chronic inflammation. (17) (18) What's interesting, though, is the effect this inflammation has on the temple wiring system.

When something in the body has gone awry (an injury, etc.)—or there's a foreign invader (like a toxin, allergen, etc.)—the immune system sends out substances called cytokines, that help fix the problem. They do this by stimulating inflammation in the body.

The problem is, cytokines that enter the bloodstream can be transported to the brain, where they signal microglia cells (brain and spinal cord cells that clean up dead neurons). Cytokines tell microglia there's a problem, which signals them to attack. Normally, this is a good thing. But if it's the ongoing consumption of an unhealthy fat stimulating this reaction (and not a virus or injury), the microglia will continuously be in attack mode. This overstimulation then can cause neurons to die, speeding up brain degeneration.

This neuroinflammation is like over-heating the electrical panel in your house. If it gets too hot, a fire could erupt which could damage the panel (or in this case, damage neurons.)

Additionally, it's been found that major depression is associated with high circulating levels of proinflammatory cytokines. And cytokines are also known to block the brain from receiving the hormone leptin which tells the body it's full and can stop eating.

I hope now you are starting to see the importance of choosing *healthy* fats, not just *any* fats. I cannot stress it enough: tracking fat consumption is more than just a number. It may sound like a lot now, but again, I encourage you to jot down notes from this chapter in the *Rebuilding Your Temple Workbook*.

References:

(1) https://hypertextbook.com/facts/2001/JacquelineLing.shtml
(2) Instituto Gulbenkian de Ciencia. "Making fat mice lean: Novel immune cells control neurons responsible for fat breakdown." ScienceDaily. ScienceDaily, 9 October 2017. www.sciencedaily.com/releases/2017/10/171009123158.htm
(3) www.mdpi.com/1422-0067/17/4/450/pdf
(4) https://nutritionandmetabolism.biomedcentral.com/articles/10.1186/1743-7075-4-3

(5) https://tim.blog/2009/06/06/saturated-fat/ or *The 6-Week Cure for the Middle-Aged Middle: The Simple Plan to Flatten Your Belly Fast!* by Michael R. Eades and Mary Dan Eades; Harmony Books, an imprint of the Crown Publishing Group; First Edition, September 8, 2009

(6) https://drhyman.com/blog/2016/03/30/fat-what-i-got-wrong-what-i-got-right/

(7) https://drhyman.com/blog/2016/05/05/fatty-liver-is-more-dangerous-than-you-might-realize-heres-how-to-heal-it/

(8) https://www.westonaprice.org/health-topics/know-your-fats/saturated-fats-and-the-lungs/

(9) https://articles.mercola.com/sites/articles/archive/2011/09/01/enjoy-saturated-fats-theyre-good-for-you.aspx

(10) https://www.ncbi.nlm.nih.gov/pubmed/20071648?dopt=AbstractPlus

(11) https://www.ncbi.nlm.nih.gov/pubmed/20685950?dopt=AbstractPlus

(12) https://www.sciencedaily.com/releases/2009/05/090529183250.htm

(13) https://www.worldhealth.net/news/omega-3-deficiency-kills-96000-americans-annually/

(14) https://lpi.oregonstate.edu/mic/other-nutrients/essential-fatty-acids

(15) https://www21.corecommerce.com/~bioage/files/astaxanthin%20800%20times%20stronger%20than%20CoQ10.pdf

(16) https://www.ncbi.nlm.nih.gov/pubmed/17638133

(17) https://www.ncbi.nlm.nih.gov/pubmed/15051604

(18) https://www.ncbi.nlm.nih.gov/pubmed/27142741

Chapter 6: Nutrients and Neurotoxins

Disclaimer: These statements have not been evaluated by the Food and Drug Administration. None of the information in this book is intended to diagnose, treat, cure, or prevent any disease. All information contained in this chapter and this book are for educational purposes only and are not intended to replace the advice of a medical doctor. Stacy Malesiewski is not a doctor and does not give medical advice, prescribe medication, or diagnose illness. Stacy is a certified health coach, journalist, and an independent Plexus ambassador. These are her personal beliefs and are not the beliefs of Plexus Worldwide, Gray Matter Media, Inc., or any other named professionals in this book. If you have a medical condition or health concern, it is advised that you see your physician immediately. It is also recommended that you consult your doctor before implementing any new health strategy or taking any new supplements. Results may vary.

The brain is probably one of the most nutritionally sensitive areas of the body. So, in addition to feeding it healthy fats and omegas, it's also important to choose foods with brain-boosting nutrients. Let's look at what I consider to be the big top four.

#1: The B Vitamins

Some of the most essential nutrients for brain health are B vitamins. B vitamins play a critical role in the formation and preservation of myelin sheath, the insulation around nerve cells that we talked about in the last chapter. According to new research, vitamin B deficiencies can result in severe myelin degeneration. (1) Without this insulation, nerve signals won't be as strong. Damaged myelin then can lead to problems with motor skills, mood, and cognitive abilities. It can even lead to serious diseases such as multiple sclerosis (MS) and Alzheimer's Disease. In fact, studies show that high doses of B-vitamins can slow brain shrinkage by as much as sevenfold, in areas specifically vulnerable to Alzheimer's disease. (2)

If that wasn't enough, B vitamins are essential for the metabolism of carbohydrates (brain fuel), and they are needed for the production of neurotransmitters, like dopamine and serotonin. Neurotransmitters are brain chemicals that transmit messages back and forth between nerve cells, communicating all sorts of information related to a variety of bodily functions, such as sleep, mood, fear, appetite, breathing, etc. But B vitamins are needed for this to happen, and unfortunately, many of us are not getting enough of them. (I will talk about the reasons why in future chapters.)

That being said, please don't go out and buy a bottle of cheap B vitamins at the drugstore. There are some things you need to know before shopping. Research suggests that approximately half of the population (maybe even 60% of us) have what's called an MTHFR gene mutation, passed down from our parents. What is that? It sounds like a swear word, but it means that half the population lacks a critical enzyme needed to make specific B vitamins "usable" in the body. Some research even suggests an MTHFR mutation is present in 98% of those with autism. (34) And most people don't even realize they have this gene mutation.

Here's how it works. When we consume folic acid (vitamin B9) we first have to convert it into Dihydrofolate (DHF), then Tetrahydrofolate (THF), and then finally into L-methylfolate (5-MTHF) for the body to be able to use it. Once it's in 5-MTHF form, though, it's all good… B9 can be moved into cells, tissues, even across the blood-brain barrier to do all its important work.

People with the MTHFR gene mutation, though, cannot complete the final step very well, which converts folic acid to the active form 5-MTHF, or L-methylfolate. So, they could be taking high doses of folic acid every single day, but still might not have enough _usable_ B9 in their system because they can't convert it.

But don't worry, you're not doomed if you have the MTHFR gene mutation. You just need to make sure you are taking vitamins that are methylated. Methylated means they're already in a usable form and active, which is necessary if you have the gene mutation.

This is why Plexus XFactor Plus™ can be beneficial (especially for those with mood, anxiety, and digestive issues). xFactor Plus™ has the most-bioactive and most-bioavailable forms of vitamins, for better absorption, including the already methylated and usable form of B9, L-methylfolate. That means even those with an MTHFR gene mutation can utilize it. If you are already taking a supplement that says it contains "folic acid" and you suspect you might have this gene mutation, I highly suggest switching to a methylated form like xFactor Plus™. Otherwise, you might just be flushing your money down the toilet (quite literally, as unused B vitamins often are secreted via urine.)

#2: Antioxidants

We've all heard of antioxidants, but what do they do exactly, and why are they important? It comes down to what's called oxidation. When an oxygen molecule in the body splits, electrons can become unpaired. When they are no longer in pairs, they become "unstable." These unstable molecules are called free radicals, and they can be super destructive. They prowl around the body looking for electrons to pair with, trying to steal them from other atoms. In the process, they can damage cells, DNA, and proteins.

Oxidation is normal, though, really—and so are free radicals. It's impossible not to make free radicals. They're produced when the body metabolizes oxygen. Cells make thousands of these free radicals naturally every day when food is burned for energy, even when we exercise. We make considerably more free radicals when we eat trans fats, pesticides, and drink excessive amounts of alcohol. And we are also exposed to them through environmental factors like pollution and radiation.

In some cases, free radicals are good because they can help fight off pathogens. But when there are too many of them for too long, it can turn into what's known as oxidative stress. This is when numerous free radicals cause a widespread and damaging domino effect in the body, leading to premature aging and disease.

That's where antioxidants come in. Antioxidants do as the name suggests. They are "anti-oxidation molecules." They are like a defense mechanism against these unstable scoundrels. They can give an electron to an unpaired free radical and remain stable themselves. They kind of "offset" them. The free radical then becomes stabilized and less destructive, which prevents the negative chain of reactions from occurring. Basically, oxidative stress occurs only when there are more free radicals roaming the body then there are antioxidants to keep them in check. Again, it comes down to balance. (Are you starting to see how important balance is to the body?)

Now, what does all this have to do with the temple wiring system?

Well, because of its high metabolic activity, the brain uses enormous amounts of oxygen, and as I mentioned, free radicals are produced when the body metabolizes oxygen. The more oxygen that is used means more free radicals are potentially produced.

What's more, as the brain ages, it becomes increasingly more difficult for nerve cells to protect themselves against free radicals, so they are especially vulnerable to damage (most often seen in memory issues). Multiple studies confirm this—that free radicals have a direct impact on brain aging (4) and even brain damage. (5)

Therefore, I cannot stress enough about the importance of antioxidants when it comes to rebuilding the temple wiring system. The most common antioxidants are beta-carotene, lutein, lycopene, selenium, vitamin A, vitamin C, and vitamin E.

Vitamin E, though, is one of the most powerful. It's the most abundant and bioavailable antioxidant in human tissues—and it is vital to the central nervous system. One study showed rodents who were fed diets lacking vitamin E developed neuromuscular problems. But then, when they were given large doses of vitamin E, these deficits were amended, and issues reversed. (6) Several other studies followed this study, showing vitamin E deficiency is linked with motor problems in humans also (but again, symptoms were reversed by vitamin E supplementation.) (7)

Other studies have shown that patients with Alzheimer's Disease often have low levels of alpha-tocopherol (a form of vitamin E) in the brain (8), and dietary intake of antioxidants can lower the risk of developing Alzheimer's Disease (vitamin E being the most protective antioxidant against Alzheimer's). (9)

The importance of these is yet another reason why I recommend Plexus XFactor Plus™ to clients. xFactor Plus™ contains 100% of the Daily Value of the most-bioactive and most-bioavailable forms of vitamins A, C, and E, as well as 150% of the Daily Value of selenium.

#3: Flavonoids

Flavonoids are a group of plant chemicals (also known as polyphenols) found in almost all fruits and vegetables, as well as roots and flowers. They are the pigments that give plants their color, and they serve as a natural insecticide and fungicide for the plant. They're exceptionally high in foods like berries, apples, citrus fruits, plums, broccoli, sweet peppers, spinach, herbal teas, cocoa, and red wine.

In humans, flavonoids are anti-inflammatory and act as antioxidants. They're basically one of the reasons why fruits and veggies are so good for you. But flavonoids aren't your typical antioxidants, especially when it comes to brain health, because they do far more than just address free radicals.

Flavonoids have been found to protect neurons from neurotoxins (which I'll discuss later in this chapter). They can reduce the risk of cardiovascular disease. They can suppress neuroinflammation, promote memory and cognitive function, as well as encourage peripheral and cerebral blood flow, which may lead to new nerve cell growth in the hippocampus. (10) Flavonoids help increase the number of connections between neurons and can also inhibit the development of amyloid plaque that is typically found in Alzheimer's patients.

For this reason, it can be very beneficial to the temple wiring system to increase the consumption of flavonoids, especially those listed above. Ideally, one should have between 5-9 servings of raw, organic fruits and veggies a day, depending on your size and gender. But, if this is not possible for you (or you feel you need more because of oxidative stress or cognitive decline), then you might need to fill in the gaps by supplementing. In this case, I once again recommend taking Plexus XFactor Plus™.

xFactor Plus™ also contains 400 mg of polyphenols. Among these are flavonoids from apple fruit extract, cranberry fruit powder, resveratrol extract, and blackcurrant fruit extract. xFactor Plus also contains grape seed extract, which is a mix of flavonoids, Vitamin E, and phenolic procyanidins (said to be 20 times higher in vitamin E and 50 times higher in vitamin C). (11) Grape seed extract also has a "vitamin E sparing" effect, so it helps you keep and better utilize the vitamin E you already have. (12)

#4: Magnesium

In my opinion, magnesium is one of the most underestimated nutrients out there, as it is involved in over 300 biochemical reactions in the body! Magnesium affects things like blood pressure, metabolism, immune function, the nervous system, and the brain... but it's been estimated by some that 90% of Americans are magnesium deficient to some degree.

I believe there are many reasons for this. One, plants typically high in magnesium (like spinach) get magnesium from the soil. And these days, the soil is often depleted of magnesium, so plants are also depleted. If they aren't depleted, then things like pesticides make it difficult for plants to absorb magnesium from the soil. In either case, it's been estimated that you now have to eat around 8 cups of organic spinach to get the same amount of nutrients your grandparents ate in just 1 cup of spinach.

Two, stress depletes magnesium. The more stressed you are, the less magnesium you're likely to retain. (I'll talk much more about this in later chapters.) Three, things like sugar, caffeine, antacids, and alcohol deplete magnesium also. Even fluoride and chlorine (in drinking water) bind to magnesium and make it less available to cells. According to medical professionals like Tana Amen BSN, RN (wife of psychiatrist, Dr. Daniel Amen, director of Amen Clinics) some medications can also strip magnesium from the body—like birth control pills, estrogen replacement therapy, blood pressure and cholesterol-lowering drugs, and diuretics (water pills). (14)

Four, magnesium and calcium need to be balanced, ideally, 1:1, because they have opposite functions. For example, calcium contracts muscles, magnesium relaxes muscles. The problem is: it's easy to get calcium by eating dairy—foods like cheese, yogurt, etc. —but magnesium, on the other hand, is a bit more difficult, as I mentioned.

Too much calcium and not enough magnesium can lead to problems like the calcification of arteries, which can lead to coronary problems like heart attack and heart disease. (That's why many heart attack patients get injections of magnesium chloride when they get to the hospital.)

Low magnesium can also lead to things like to mitral valve prolapse, muscle spasms and cramps, high blood pressure/hypertension, hormone problems, sleep/energy problems, and poor bone health.

In terms of the temple wiring system, magnesium also plays a vital role in how the brain learns. You see, when we think, information is sent back and forth through pathways in the brain, in the spaces between neurons. Learning *new* things involves forming *new* pathways. When we learn something new, we are essentially rewiring the brain with a new connection to understand, move, or remember something. This happens because of brain plasticity. It's the flexibility and pliability of the brain that allows these new pathways to form. A rigid brain will have a difficult time creating new pathways.

What does this have to do with magnesium? Well, studies show that magnesium can enhance brain plasticity. (13) It also enhances synaptic transmission, because magnesium hangs out in in the space between neurons, making sure things like calcium and glutamate don't over-stimulate receptors, which can lead to cell death and neuron damage. (I'll talk more about this later in this chapter, too.)

What's more, data suggests magnesium may protect against chronic pain, stroke, and anxiety. (15) In fact, one study showed that magnesium-deficient mice displayed increased anxiety-like behavior (16), and another showed low magnesium in humans was associated with depression. (17) But, a separate study showed that consuming just 248 mg of magnesium daily for six weeks *improved* depression scores. (18)

Maybe at this point, you're considering getting some lab work done to determine if you are magnesium deficient. Unfortunately, it's not that simple. Magnesium levels are hard to measure. Most magnesium is stored in bones, some of it is in cells, but only a small amount resides in the blood—which is what conventional labs use to test magnesium levels. So, in my experience, these tests are often inaccurate.

Again, it is imperative that you discuss these concerns with your doctor—especially if you are taking any medications. Do not just start taking magnesium on your own, as magnesium can interfere with certain OTC and prescription drugs. If your doctor has approved magnesium supplementation, though, I love Plexus Bio Cleanse™. (But again, you will want to get your doctor's approval first as magnesium can interfere with some medications.)

Bio Cleanse™ not only has 380 mg of magnesium hydroxide per serving, but it also has 150 mg of vitamin C (250% of the daily recommended value) for antioxidant support, and 50 mg of a bioflavonoid complex containing orange (peel), lemon (peel) and quince (whole fruit).

Neurotoxins

Because the brain is so nutritionally sensitive, these nutrients can be extremely beneficial for the temple wiring system. However, being _so_ sensitive is _not_ good when it comes to things like food additives and chemicals… especially those chemicals that neurosurgeon, Dr. Russel Blaylock, calls neurotoxins or excitotoxins. The big two that I personally stay far (FAR) away from are monosodium glutamate (MSG) and aspartame (NutraSweet and Equal).

Let's start with MSG.

What is monosodium glutamate? Well, glutamate is an amino acid (a building block of protein). It's also a neurotransmitter. It's an "amino acid neurotransmitter"—essentially, it's an amino acid that can transmit a message via a nerve synapse. Therefore, it's what's known as an _excitatory_ neurotransmitter because it "excites" or "stimulates" nerve cells to communicate messages.

So, glutamate is not a bad thing. It's found naturally in plant and animal protein foods like tomatoes, cheese, fish, and mushrooms, and the body can produce it on its own. In fact, glutamate is the most abundant neurotransmitter in the body and is especially prevalent in the brain.

So why do I stay away from MSG then, if glutamate is such a good thing? Well, first, glutamate and MSG are not the same. Monosodium glutamate (MSG) is manufactured with only the sodium salt of glutamate. And because it's manufactured it is a synthetic form, containing byproducts and contaminants. It is also what's known as "free glutamate," meaning it has been freed from other amino acids.

Why is this a problem? Because "bound glutamate" is an unchanged protein source, so it digests slowly. Remember the analogy of rollercoaster carbs versus Sunday drive carbs at the beginning of this book? Well, it's similar to free and bound glutamate. Free glutamate digests very quickly—_too_ quickly, causing massive spikes in the amount of glutamate in the blood. This is not a good thing because cells have glutamate receptors, and remember, glutamate is a _stimulant_ for nerve cells (and we all know what happens when we consume too much of a stimulant).

According to Dr. Blaylock, excitotoxins like MSG _over_-stimulate neuron receptors. The neurons fire impulses over and over again. They fire them so fast that they become exhausted to the point that the neurons die after about one hour, according to Blaylock. (19) Other research confirms this. (20) This cell death takes place in parts of the brain that control things like behavior, emotions, the onset of puberty, sleep cycles, immunity, and metabolism. (For an in-depth look at this, I _highly_ recommend Dr. Blaylock's book, _Excitotoxins: The Taste That Kills,_ available on Amazon.com.)

Perhaps you're wondering why MSG would even be added to food then. Well, because it makes food taste better. It stimulates cells in the tongue as well as the brain, so they are used as "flavor enhancers."

Some argue that the blood-brain barrier (which protects the brain from unwanted and harmful substances) protects the brain from neurotoxins like MSG. However, research confirms that inflammation can cause openings in the blood-brain barrier, allowing things like neurotoxins to enter. (21) Therefore, people with chronic inflammation (as seen in things like gut issues, arthritis, allergies, infections, pain, and depression) could be more at risk for neurotoxin damage.

Regardless, many health issues have been linked to regular consumption of MSG: obesity, eye damage, headaches/migraines, fatigue and disorientation, and depression. It's also been referred to as "MSG Symptom Complex" and can involve symptoms such as numbness, burning sensation, tingling, facial pressure or tightness, chest pain or difficulty breathing, headache, nausea, rapid heartbeat, drowsiness, and weakness. (22)

According to Dr. Blaylock, MSG can potentially trigger or worsen learning disabilities, Alzheimer's disease, Parkinson's disease, Lou Gehrig's disease, and more. (23) (24)

While MSG is typically just thought of as an ingredient in Chinese food, it's found in thousands of other foods, too, especially processed foods and restaurant food. It can be in things like crackers, baby food/formula, deli meats, salad dressings, frozen dinners, and canned soups.

Despite all this, MSG is still widely used, and most people have no idea they're eating it. Why? Because MSG is sometimes called by other names. Below is a comprehensive list published by popular osteopathic physician and NY Times Bestselling author, Dr. Mercola, on his website at mercola.com. (25) (His article on the subject is highly recommended also.)

Ingredients that ALWAYS contain MSG (According to Dr. Mercola):

- Monosodium Glutamate
- Hydrolyzed Vegetable Protein
- Hydrolyzed Protein
- Hydrolyzed Plant Protein
- Plant Protein Extract
- Sodium Caseinate
- Calcium Caseinate
- Yeast Extract
- Yeast Nutrient
- Monopotassium Glutamate
- Textured Protein
- Autolyzed Yeast
- Hydrolyzed Oat Flour

Ingredients that OFTEN contain MSG or create MSG during processing (According to Dr. Mercola):

- Flavors and Flavorings
- Seasonings
- Natural Flavors and Flavorings
- Natural Pork Flavoring
- Natural Beef Flavoring
- Natural Chicken Flavoring
- Soy Sauce
- Soy Protein Isolate
- Soy Protein
- Bouillon
- Stock
- Broth
- Malt Extract
- Malt Flavoring
- Barley Malt
- Anything Enzyme Modified
- Carrageenan
- Maltodextrin
- Pectin
- Enzymes
- Protease

- Corn Starch
- Citric Acid
- Powdered Milk
- Anything Protein Fortified
- Anything Ultra-Pasteurized

The Electrical Box

While MSG can potentially cause many unwanted side effects, one of the most concerning (to me) is that animal studies suggest it may also cause lesions on the hypothalamus. (26) What is the hypothalamus? It's a part of the brain that makes hormones that help regulate hunger and thirst, as well as other things like body temperature, sex drive, emotional responses, heart rate, blood pressure, electrolyte balance, and circadian rhythm (basically your internal clock that regulates your sleep/wake cycle.) Simply put, the hypothalamus is a vital part of the Autonomic Nervous System that communicates with the endocrine system.

Like an electrical box in your home that is linked to many different outlets and appliances throughout a house, the brain is connected to many different organs and glands in the temple of the body. The Hypothalamus is an area of the brain that acts as a sort of circuit breaker. When electricity comes into your home, it usually is divided into circuits. A circuit breaker senses how much current is needed. It is the "stop-and-go" switch that will either allow the current to keep moving or "trip" the power to stop the flow.

The hypothalamus works similarly, but it senses the body's need for hormones. It essentially makes "stop-and-go" hormones that either keep hormone production moving or it "trips" production to stop hormone production.

For example, if we look at appetite, the hypothalamus balances our food intake with our energy requirements. It senses how much fat, glucose, and insulin we have in the blood. It senses how much leptin and ghrelin we have (hunger hormones that say when we should eat and when we should stop eating). It takes all this information and uses it to communicate with the liver, intestines, kidneys, even fat tissue to coordinate metabolism.

This is just one example, but the hypothalamus communicates with many other areas of the body like the pituitary gland, thyroid, adrenal glands, and kidneys, among other things.

Now, if MSG can potentially cause lesions on the hypothalamus, think about how many different bodily processes this could theoretically affect. Think about how many appliances and outlets would be affected in your house if the electrical box had faulty circuit breakers. Therefore, as you attempt to rebuild the temple wiring system, it might be advantageous to remove MSG and other excitotoxins from your diet—especially if you are already experiencing symptoms of MSG Symptom Complex. As always, these concerns should be discussed with your doctor.

I know this can seem daunting. There are so many "code words" out there. But the easiest way to ensure you are not eating MSG (or other excitotoxins) is to eat food closest to its natural form. Avoid boxed, bagged, and canned foods and start cooking and eating real food! Eat natural cuts of organic meat, not processed meats like sausage, hot dogs, and deli meats. Or if you do eat those meats, natural, uncured bacon and organic, cage-free chicken sausage may be a better option.

This is especially important for those who adopt a ketogenic diet. So many people think that eating a high-fat diet means they can load up on bacon, sausage, and other processed meats full of excitotoxins. Yes, you might stay in a state of fat-burning eating those things—and you may even lose weight at first—but it may also come at a very high cost to your wiring system.

Sweet Excitotoxicity

The other neurotoxin that I personally stay _far_ away from is aspartame—a low-calorie, artificial sweetener (200 times sweeter than sugar) that is typically sold under the brand names NutraSweet® and Equal®. Aspartame, like MSG, contains natural amino acids in a very unnatural fashion.

Aspartame contains the amino acids L-aspartic acid and L-phenylalanine, which, like glutamate, are also excitatory, so they produce the same stimulating effects. However, these two amino acids are naturally present in foods like meat and eggs in minimal quantities (typically less than 5%) and with other amino acids, so the stimulation is controlled.

In aspartame, however, the ratio is closer to 50% L-phenylalanine and 40% L-aspartic acid. What's the other 10%? Wood alcohol. This is an unnatural amount that the body simply was not designed to handle. Studies show the excess of phenylalanine in aspartame can lead to reduced levels of dopamine and serotonin, and the excessive levels of aspartic acid can lead to the deterioration of astrocytes (cells in the central nervous system) and neurons. (28) Aspartame is also known to contribute to the formation of tumors in the central nervous system. (28)

What's more, upon ingestion, aspartame is broken down, converted, and oxidized into formaldehyde in various tissues, which has been associated with migraines in testing. (29) Other aspartame-induced symptoms can include fatigue, anxiety, depression, sleep disturbances, and abdominal pain.

So how do you stay away from aspartame? First be wary of processed foods that claim to be sugar-free, "diet," or low or no-calorie (*especially* diet soda!). These types of products often contain aspartame. Therefore, it's important to read labels... or better yet, just eat real food.

Pain, Tingling, and Numbness... Oh My!

Care for the temple wiring system isn't solely about brain health. It's also important to consider the outside or "peripheral" nerves that carry messages from the brain to the rest of the body (and back again). Sometimes these nerves can become damaged or diseased from things like diabetes, physical injury, alcoholism, a sedentary lifestyle, or autoimmune conditions. This can result in what's called peripheral neuropathy, which can result in symptoms like pain, tingling, numbness, cramping, muscle weakness, over-sensitivity, even lack of coordination.

These are symptoms that should not be taken lightly and should be discussed with your doctor immediately. You may even want to ask your physician about taking Plexus Nerve™. Plexus Nerve™ is a combination of vitamins, minerals, herbs, and amino acids to help support healthy nerve cells and nervous system.

Some of the ingredients that I love most about Plexus Nerve™ are:

- Acetyl L-Carnitine (ALC): ALC is an amino acid that is naturally produced in the body. It has been shown to decrease pain, increase nerve regeneration, and even vibratory perception. Both animal and human data consistently demonstrate the neuroprotective and antinociceptive effects of ALC. (30)
- Horse Chestnut Extract: This is an extract from the Aesculus hippocastanum tree bark. It has been used as a traditional remedy for arthritis and joint pain for centuries and is useful in addressing mild to moderate blood flow disorder. Because horse chestnut can lower blood sugar, though, you must discuss this with your doctor before taking Horse Chestnut Extract, especially if you have diabetes. It can also interfere with some medications used to treat bipolar disorder.
- Butcher's Broom: Butcher's Broom (Ruscus aculeatus) is a small evergreen shrub. One study shows Butcher's Broom strengthens blood vessels, reduces capillary fragility, and helps maintain healthy circulation. It also reduces venous capacity and pooling of blood in the legs and exerts protective effects on capillaries, the vascular endothelium, and smooths muscle. The study also notes that Butcher's Broom can alleviate the worsening effects of orthostatic hypotension in environmentally hot conditions. (31)

- Quercetin: Quercetin is a common flavonoid found in many fresh fruits and vegetables. Its antioxidant properties affect the cardiovascular system, inflammation, and can help with stress. It's also been found to be anti-atherogenic, and anti-carcinogenic, and animal studies indicate that QC treatment has nerve growth-promoting effects. (32)

Aside from Plexus Nerve™, I do not know of any other therapy that can help the body generate Nerve Growth Factor (NGF)—the only peptide that can help stimulate the regeneration of damaged nerve fibers. Plexus Nerve™ also has an abundance of B vitamins as well as a smaller amount of magnesium, zinc, and copper.

Additional Pain Relief

Plexus Ease

For additional nerve pain relief or pain that is associated with inflammation, you may also want to discuss Plexus Ease® with your doctor. This product is intended to do as the name suggests: "ease" discomfort. The Ease ingredients I find most noteworthy are:

- Green-lipped mussel: This patented, green-lipped mussel is sourced from New Zealand and contains lyprinol, which is a mix of the EPA and DHA omega 3 fatty acids that I talked about in the last chapter. Studies show green-lipped mussel has substantial anti-inflammatory properties (33) and lyprinol can provide pain relief for patients with osteoarthritis. (34) However, DO NOT take this product if you have a shellfish allergy.
- Bromelain: An enzyme found in pineapples that helps digest protein. It also is anti-inflammatory (especially regarding allergies, sinusitis, and asthma) and it assists with pain, especially following surgery and pain associated with osteoarthritis and rheumatoid arthritis. (35)
- Serrapeptase: This is an enzyme that breaks down fibrin, which is a blood protein involved in coagulation, clotting, and formation of arterial plaque. Studies also show that serrapeptase has substantial anti-inflammatory properties, especially when it comes to post-surgery swelling. (36)
- Turmeric: Turmeric contains curcumin. Studies show curcumin acts similarly to various medications, even tumor blockers (37) and exhibits antioxidant, anti-inflammatory, antiviral, and antifungal properties. (38) There currently are over 10,000 peer-reviewed articles on turmeric.

CBD

The issue of pain and inflammation leads me to another very hotly-discussed topic these days: CBD. I'm sure you have heard of this at some point (unless you live under a rock). Health professionals everywhere are discussing it, and businesses everywhere are selling versions of it. But what on earth is it, and why is the world going nuts over it?

Well CBD stands for cannabidiol. It's one of 120 other compounds called cannabinoids found in the marijuana plant. The CBD compound does not cause intoxication, though. (It's the THC compound in marijuana that causes users to feel "high," _not_ the CBD compound.)

So what makes CBD so highly sought after these days?

To understand, let's go back to our discussion on the nervous system. Inside the nervous system, we have at least two kinds of cannabinoid receptors. First, there are CB1 receptors, located in the central nervous system (brain and spinal cord). Then, there are CB2 receptors, located in the peripheral nervous system (in our nerves).

Like electrical outlets, these receptors receive and bind to cannabinoid compounds that then "spark" or activate different functions in the nervous system—but not just any functions. These compounds activate functions responsible for keeping the body in balance—like a balanced appetite, temperature, inflammation, pleasure/reward, immune response, mood, and sleep, to name just a few. (39)

Once the body returns to balance, the cannabinoid compounds are broken down by enzymes, and they are removed from the body. All of these things (the cannabinoids, the receptors, and the enzymes) work together to form what is known as the endocannabinoid system.

At this point, some of you might be thinking, "*Wait! What?! We have a marijuana system in the body?!*" The answer is no... and yes. Let me explain.

The body makes its own cannabinoid compounds naturally (these are called endo-cannabinoids, "endo" meaning *"within"* the body). These are similar to the cannabinoids in the marijuana plant. This was discovered about 25 years ago when scientists were studying the effects of marijuana on various health issues. They found that our body not only makes similar compounds but that we also make enzymes for them, and have many receptors for them too. (In fact, some believe cannabinoid receptors are the most abundant receptors in the central nervous system.) Long story short, this newly-found bodily system was then named after the marijuana compounds that were being studied at the time.

Now back to the issue of pain. If we have a copious amount of these cannabinoid receptors in the nervous system, and they are involved in various nerve functions as well as the balance of inflammation, then could it stand to reason increasing cannabinoid compounds via CBD oil would decrease inflammation and thereby pain?

Research is suggesting yes, it *is* a possibility. (40)

One study found that CBD reduced the pain response of rats who underwent surgical incisions. (41) Other studies found CBD proved beneficial for arthritis (42) and osteoarthritis. (43) Another study also found that rats who received CBD orally had reduced sciatic nerve pain and inflammation. (44)

But it doesn't end there. Research also suggests cannabidiol is a potential treatment for anxiety disorders (45) even showing promise for pediatric anxiety and insomnia in posttraumatic stress disorders. (46) One study also showed CBD had antidepressant-like effects. (47)

That being said, the endocannabinoid system is still a relatively new discovery, meaning more research still needs conducted. However, the data we have thus far suggests CBD could be promising for a host of ailments. That being said, there are many different types of CBD, so it's important to discuss these with your practitioner, first, before trying any type of CBD product. In fact, this is especially true if you are taking any medications as CBD may prevent the body from metabolizing certain drugs, so they could stay in the body longer.

CBD Oils, Lotions, Capsules and Everything In Between

One of the more common forms of CBD is CBD oil. To make CBD oil, the cannabidiol compound is extracted from the plant and then diluted with a carrier oil. CBD oil comes in three forms: full spectrum, broad spectrum, and isolate. Isolate means the compound was extracted by itself without any of the other cannabinoid compounds. Full spectrum means that the oil contains *all* the other compounds (but only *trace* amounts of THC). Full spectrum CBD oil also contains flavonoids and both aromatic and essential oils. Broad spectrum is similar to full spectrum, but it does not contain any THC, not even trace amounts.

While CBD isolate is more concentrated, some believe full spectrum CBD oil is more effective because it contains all of the natural compounds of the plant that work together synergistically as nature intended. In my experience it is usually dependent upon the user.

CBD also comes in topical lotions, capsules, gummies, and sprays. It also comes in edible liquid forms such as tinctures or concentrates. A tincture is squirted by drops into the mouth with a dropper. Concentrates are also, but they are placed under the tongue. Concentrates also come in much stronger doses, and are probably not ideal for CBD beginners.

Hemp and CBD

Another type of CBD product is hemp oil. Hemp is sometimes mistaken for marijuana, but it is not the same. Technically, both hemp and marijuana come from the same *Cannabis sativa* species, but they are different plants altogether. The hemp plant contains little or no THC (less than .3%), whereas the marijuana plant (also called cannabis) contains significantly more THC (between 5-35%). Therefore, hemp cannot get a person "high" like marijuana/cannibis can.

That being said, hemp contains high levels of beneficial CBD, though, which is why many CBD products come from the hemp plant. It is important to choose a quality brand, though, because not all hemp or CBD products are created equal.

A quality product should always say how much CBD is in the product and if other ingredients were added. It should also state the lab tested for contaminants and quality. This is not always done so it is important to read labels.

I'm excited to announce that Plexus will be releasing it's own hemp extract oil and cannabidiol isolate oil coming this fall (2019). Stay tuned for more information on that.

** Note: CBD vape oil is also available some places. However, it is not recommended because these also contain propylene glycol which, when burned, can rturn into formaldehyde.

References

(1) https://www.ncbi.nlm.nih.gov/pubmed/28875857
(2) https://www.ncbi.nlm.nih.gov/pubmed/23690582
(3) https://www.ncbi.nlm.nih.gov/pubmed/12872680
(4) https://www.ncbi.nlm.nih.gov/pubmed/15182885
(5) https://www.ncbi.nlm.nih.gov/pubmed/2701375
(6) https://www.ncbi.nlm.nih.gov/pubmed/20187127
(7) https://www.ncbi.nlm.nih.gov/pmc/articles/PMC4276978/#B24-nutrients-06-05453
(8) https://www.ncbi.nlm.nih.gov/pubmed/21504121
(9) https://www.ncbi.nlm.nih.gov/pubmed/22543848
(10) https://www.ncbi.nlm.nih.gov/pubmed/19685255

(11) https://www.liebertpub.com/doi/abs/10.1089/109662003772519831
(12) https://www.ncbi.nlm.nih.gov/pmc/articles/PMC4288794/
(13) https://www.ncbi.nlm.nih.gov/pubmed/20152124
(14) https://tanaamen.com/2013/04/23/magnesium-a-marvelously-powerful-health-booster/
(15) https://www.ncbi.nlm.nih.gov/pubmed/29882776
(16) https://www.ncbi.nlm.nih.gov/pubmed/21835188
(17) http://www.jabfm.org/content/28/2/249.long
(18) https://journals.plos.org/plosone/article?id=10.1371/journal.pone.0180067
(19) https://youtu.be/tTSvlGniHok
(20) https://www.ncbi.nlm.nih.gov/pmc/articles/PMC2802046/
(21) https://www.sciencedaily.com/releases/2014/06/140602104749.htm
(22) https://www.ncbi.nlm.nih.gov/pubmed/9215242
(23) Excitotoxins: The Taste That Kills by Russell L. Blaylock
(24) https://www.ncbi.nlm.nih.gov/pmc/articles/PMC5421223/
(25) https://articles.mercola.com/sites/articles/archive/2009/04/21/msg-is-this-silent-killer-lurking-in-your-kitchen-cabinets.aspx
(26) https://www.sciencedirect.com/science/article/pii/0006899384910631
(27) https://www.ncbi.nlm.nih.gov/pmc/articles/PMC2610632/
(28) https://www.ncbi.nlm.nih.gov/pubmed/23553132
(29) https://www.ncbi.nlm.nih.gov/pubmed/18627677
(30) https://www.naturalmedicinejournal.com/journal/2010-08/therapeutic-effects-acetyl-l-carnitine-peripheral-neuropathy-review-literature
(31) https://www.ncbi.nlm.nih.gov/pubmed/11152059
(32) https://www.ncbi.nlm.nih.gov/pubmed/22183523
(33) https://www.sciencedirect.com/science/article/pii/S1096495907001522
(34) https://www.ncbi.nlm.nih.gov/pubmed/12872680
(35) https://www.ncbi.nlm.nih.gov/pmc/articles/PMC3529416/
(36) https://www.ncbi.nlm.nih.gov/pubmed/6366808
(37) https://www.ncbi.nlm.nih.gov/pubmed/17569205
(38) https://www.ncbi.nlm.nih.gov/pubmed/12676044
(39) https://www.ncbi.nlm.nih.gov/pubmed/19675519
(40) https://www.ncbi.nlm.nih.gov/pmc/articles/PMC5922297/
(41) https://www.ncbi.nlm.nih.gov/pmc/articles/PMC5478794/
(42) https://www.ncbi.nlm.nih.gov/pmc/articles/PMC4851925/
(43) https://insights.ovid.com/crossref?an=00006396-201712000-00018
(44) https://www.ncbi.nlm.nih.gov/pubmed/17157290
(45) https://www.ncbi.nlm.nih.gov/pubmed/26341731
(46) https://www.ncbi.nlm.nih.gov/pmc/articles/PMC5101100
(47) https://www.ncbi.nlm.nih.gov/pubmed/24923339

Phase 3:

Rebuilding the Framework

Materials: Organic Beef, Poultry, Dairy, Eggs, Quinoa, Buckwheat, and Lentils

Tools: Plexus Lean™

Chapter 7: Good Protein, Bad Protein

Congratulations on completing Phase 2 of the temple rebuild!! Now that we've covered the fueling and wiring systems, it's time to move on to Phase 3: the "framework." In this phase, we will talk a lot about protein. Proteins are made up of amino acids, which are like the building blocks of the body. They help to build muscle, blood, internal organs, hair, and nails. They are also important building blocks of bones, muscles, cartilage, and skin. They are used to build and repair tissue too. They come together to form our structure, like the framework of a house, which supports the entire body.

But... that's not all. You also need protein to make enzymes, hormones, and other body chemicals too. And as I mentioned in Phase 1, protein is also important for keeping blood sugars steady. Unlike carbohydrates and fats, though, your body can't store protein. It has no protein "stash" to pull from if you run low. So, it's important that you eat enough protein every single day.

And yes, if you are on the standard ketogenic diet, you may only be eating approximately 15% of your total calories from protein. So, maybe you're thinking, *"It's only 15%. Does it matter that much?"* But only eating 15%, is precisely WHY I'm stressing the importance of it. If you aren't eating that much of it, you need to make it count.

There's good protein, and then there's "not so good" protein when it comes to rebuilding your temple. There's even what I'd consider _bad_ protein. Most people don't consider the kinds of protein, but it's extremely important. Think of it this way: you wouldn't use rotten or warped boards to frame your house, would you? You wouldn't use cheap boards either, right? Right. You wouldn't do this because you want your house to be strong, sturdy, and able to withstand the elements for years to come.

Why then would you choose substandard and cheap proteins? You should want your body's structure to be strong and sturdy, too. You should want it to be able to withstand the elements for years to come also. Therefore, over the next few pages, we will be talking a lot about protein and other factors that are involved in rebuilding the framework of the temple.

Calculating Protein

As I mentioned before, when you are using carbs (glucose) for fuel, protein can be converted to glycogen and used like glucose, through a process called gluconeogenesis. This can even happen on the ketogenic diet too if you do not get enough fats for energy and you overindulge in protein. This could kick you out of a state of ketosis and even cause you to lose muscle.

The good news is, over time, most people become fat-adapted on the keto diet, meaning fat-fuel becomes a habit for their body, and so do not need as much protein after time. While in a state of ketosis, the body experiences an increase in circulating leucine, which is a branched amino acid that helps *preserve* lean body mass and can increase protein synthesis in muscles.

Because it's such a fine line, though (between too much protein and not enough), some people develop a "protein fear" on the ketogenic diet, and they severely restrict protein to make sure they stay in ketosis. But, this is the WRONG way to do it, in my opinion.

I've seen both keto and non-keto dieters limit protein to such an extent that their hair starts feeling rough, their nails start feeling brittle, and they start losing muscle mass or experiencing muscle weakness. I've seen people with increased swelling in their legs, feet, and ankles. (Protein is involved in keeping fluid from collecting in tissue.) I've even seen people sabotage their thyroid and other hormones by neglecting this critical part of a healthy diet. (See bullet points below for more info.)

Regardless of whether you're using glucose or ketones for fuel, protein is absolutely crucial for optimal health—especially if you're trying to lose weight because it affects the metabolic rate. Without enough protein, the body burns calories much slower causing excess fat to be *stored*, not *burned*. Think of it this way: the lower your protein intake is, the lower your metabolic rate is. The higher your protein intake is, the higher your metabolic rate is (staying within your allotted macros, of course).

Speaking of allotted macros... how much do we need? Some guidelines state that women need 46 grams of protein each day, and men need 56 grams. Other sources say it should be 0.66 grams of protein for every 2 pounds of body weight.

In my opinion, these are still too general. There are other factors that should be taken into consideration also. So it's important to discuss these situations with your doctor:

- If you are exercising—lifting weights, trying to tone your body, or doing any type of high-intensity interval training—you may need more protein than the typical person, especially before and after workouts (even if you're on a keto diet).
- If you are over the age of 65, you may need to replace muscle loss from aging, and so you might need more protein too.
- If you have thyroid issues, you may need more protein as well. Protein modifies thyroid hormone levels according to body temperature. (1) In fact, a low-protein diet or insufficient intake of essential amino acids can contribute to thyroid hormone abnormalities and negatively alter the hypothalamus-pituitary-thyroid axis. (2) This is another reason why a ketogenic diet may not be suitable for thyroid patients (15% may not be adequate).
- If you have blood sugar imbalances or metabolic issues, you may need more protein to stabilize blood sugar levels. This goes for people who are stressed too, as high stress can lead to blood sugar imbalances and hypoglycemia. Chronic stress can even cause body tissue to break down, in which case you will need more protein. (I will talk more about stress in later chapters.)
- If you suffer from low dopamine levels (and have attention deficit issues like as ADD or ADHD, or mood issues like depression and anxiety), then you might need more protein because you might need more of the amino acid tyrosine. Tyrosine forms DOPA, which is then converted to dopamine, so it acts as a precursor.

Of course, there is always at least one exception to the rule. One instance where it might not be good to increase protein consumption is if you have liver disease or cirrhosis of the liver. The liver works to cleanse harmful substances from the blood—things like ammonia, which is produced during protein metabolism. ***If you have liver issues or a family history of liver issues, it is imperative to discuss this with your doctor before increasing your protein intake.***

As you can see, because of the many variables, there is no "magic number" that fits everyone when it comes to protein. It may be worthwhile to revisit chapter 3, though, and reevaluate your calculations to make sure you chose the right percentage.

Or, if you want to be *really* technical, you can confirm those numbers and make sure they fit you, by calculating your precise protein needs according to lean body mass and activity level. (I will explain how to do this in the section below, but there is an easier calculation sheet in the *Rebuilding Your Temple Workbook* also if you need help. If you are not concerned with being overly technical, you can just skip the rest of this section and move on to the next part of this chapter.)

First, let's determine your lean body mass. This is your total weight (in pounds) minus your percentage of body fat. So, the calculation looks like this:

Step 1: Weight – body fat % = lean body mass

You probably already know what you weigh. So, next, you will need to determine your percentage of body fat. You can either use a skinfold caliper to measure body fat, or you can guesstimate using the image below. Which figure looks most like you? That's your estimated percentage.

Body Fat Percentage

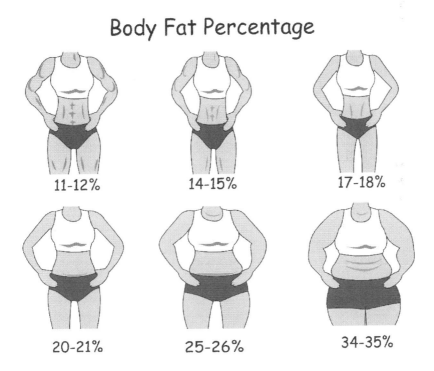

| 11-12% | 14-15% | 17-18% |

| 20-21% | 25-26% | 34-35% |

Once you've determined body fat percentage, subtract that from your total weight as indicated in step 1. This equals your lean body mass. Next, multiply your lean body mass by your activity level. The calculation looks like this:

Step 2: Lean body mass x activity level = grams of protein needed

How do you calculate your activity level? Let's think about it. If you multiply your lean body mass by 1, you will get the same amount of grams of protein as you have pounds of body mass. That's *a lot* of protein and a lot of building blocks! In order to NEED that much protein, you would have to be extremely active. So, the number 1 is considered the maximum activity level.

According to Volek and Phinney (*The Art and Science of Low Carbohydrate Performance*), it goes backward from there. If 1.0 is the maximum activity level, then .9 is high activity, .8 is moderate activity, .7 is light activity, and .6 is no activity (sedentary).

For example, a person with 120 pounds of lean body mass who does moderate activity would multiply 120 x .8, which equals 96 grams of protein per day. These calculations are a good starting point, but you may need even more if you are not on a ketogenic diet and struggle with the other factors that I mentioned earlier: blood sugar imbalances, thyroid dysfunction, or lifting weights. In these instances, you can raise that number as you and your doctor see fit. (Revisit chapter three for more info.)

If you want to see what these calculations mean in terms of percentage of calories (to compare to these calculations with those in chapter 3) simply put the protein *grams* back into protein *calories* by multiplying your protein by 4. (Remember there are four calories in each gram of protein.) For example, 96 grams of protein equals 384 protein calories. The calculation looks like this: 96 x 4 = 384.

If you have a 2,000 calorie/day allotment, then this amount of protein would equate to approximately 19% of your total calories. That calculation looks like this: 384 ÷ 2000 = .192 (converted to 19.2%). This is quite a bit higher than the standard keto 15%, but some people who have chronic stress, blood sugar imbalances, etc. can still maintain ketosis eating this much protein. But some people can't. This is why it is so important to test ketone levels to make sure.

Easing Into It

For many of you, these new protein calculations might be very different from your current protein intake. Increasing protein all of a sudden could make it difficult for the body to digest this much protein at first (especially if you have gut issues and do not make enough digestive enzymes to break it down properly. I'll talk about this more in the next phase.)

If you are concerned about this, it might be better to ease into this much protein. Maybe consider working your way up to these calculations. I personally would *not* go from eating 30 grams of protein a day to eating 100 grams a day. You probably won't feel good, and probably won't have fun in the bathroom. A better option might be to increase your protein a little bit each day until you reach your ideal number.

Another thing that I find very helpful is to mix two tablespoons of raw apple cider vinegar with 1-2 cups of water and drink the entire glass before a heavy protein meal. If you don't like the taste, I also sometimes add a dropper of liquid stevia and ice. Proteins need acids to digest, and because apple cider vinegar contains acetic acid, it can help the body break down protein into the necessary amino acids. (I'll talk more about apple cider vinegar and digestion in the next phase.) I also take Plexus® Pro Bio 5, which contains Proteases, enzymes which break down proteins. (I'll talk much more about Pro Bio 5 in later chapters, too.)

Hunger Hormones

One of the benefits of increasing protein is that it is satiating. It helps curb appetite by keeping you fuller, longer. Other factors that contribute to appetite are the hunger hormones Ghrelin and Leptin. Ghrelin is an appetite-stimulating hormone made in the stomach. It says, "eat, eat, eat!" It is what makes you feel hungry. Leptin, on the other hand, is an appetite-decreasing hormone produced in fat tissue. It says, "stop, stop, stop!" It is what helps you feel full. In simplified terms: Ghrelin increases hunger, while leptin decreases hunger.

Let's compare it to building a house or rebuilding our temple. Remember when I told you that tracking macros was like the thermostat of the house? Tracking tells us how much we fuel we need. At that time I said we need this thermostat because some things can make us feel like we _need_ more fuel than we actually do. Ghrelin and Leptin are two of those things.

Having imbalanced hunger hormones is like having a faulty front door in the winter that keeps letting in cold air. According to the thermostat, the house needs more fuel. But in reality, the house just needs a new front door that knows how to open and close at the appropriate time (or in the case of hunger hormones, eat and stop).

Both Ghrelin and Leptin are crucial factors in balancing food intake and maintaining a healthy weight. Unfortunately, these two hormones don't work efficiently for some people, as problems can arise over time. One, lack of sleep can disrupt the functioning of Ghrelin and Leptin, which is why it is not uncommon to overeat when you are tired. Also, Ghrelin is not just released in times of hunger; it is also released as a response to stress... which is why some people suffer from "stress eating." Other things can also affect hunger hormones, like chronic inflammation in the hypothalamus caused by some processed foods.

When all these factors are present for an extended period, it can alter how these hunger hormones naturally operate. For example, too much Ghrelin (which says "Eat!") can override signals sent from the GI tract that says to stop eating. Over time, some people can become Leptin resistant, which means Leptin (which says "stop!") is released, but the brain doesn't recognize it. It becomes sort of like "white noise." It's there, but not noticeable anymore. Then what you have is too much Ghrelin that says "eat," but the brain won't recognize the Leptin that says, "stop!" This creates a perfect storm for overeating and weight gain.

So, the question becomes: how do you rebuild or balance your hunger hormones? Obviously, getting enough sleep and managing stress is important, as is cutting out processed food and addressing inflammation. But another way might be to incorporate high-intensity interval training (HIIT) or burst training into your exercise routine. Steady-state cardio is an excellent form of exercise, don't get me wrong, but it increases Ghrelin and lowers Leptin (to make you hungry afterward). This could be problematic for someone who already has hunger hormone imbalances. A HIIT or burst routine (like 30-second sprints or weightlifting) on the other hand, can decrease Ghrelin (3) and increase Leptin (as well as increase the cells' sensitivity to Leptin too).

Another thing that helps balance hunger hormones is to eat more protein! Studies have shown that a high protein meal decreases Ghrelin concentrations afterward, more so than a high carbohydrate meal does. (4) For those who are trying to lose inches as well as pounds, higher protein percentages mixed with HIIT or burst training could prove to be an excellent strategy.

Choosing Complete Proteins

So now that you are starting to see the importance of protein, let's talk about the types of protein before you run out to the grocery store. Here's the basic gist: Protein as I said, is made up of amino acids. There are 20 amino acids found in the foods we need. Nine of these are called "essential amino acids" because the body NEEDS them. Just like essential fatty acids, the body cannot make these on its own, so it's "essential" that we get them from our food. (The technical names of these nine essential amino acids are: histidine, valine, isoleucine, leucine, phenylalanine, threonine, tryptophan, methionine, and lysine.)

If a food contains all nine of these essential amino acids, it's called a "complete" protein. Complete proteins are things like dairy, chicken, beef, fish, and eggs. Foods that do not have all nine essential amino acids are called "incomplete" proteins. These are things like grains, beans, nuts, and seeds. These are NOT "bad" proteins; they are just not complete, meaning they do not contain _all_ of the amino acids that we need.

Some incomplete proteins may contain some essential amino acids but do not have all nine. Or perhaps they have other "nonessential amino acids" (these are not "essential" to consume because our body can make them on its own).

So, when we talk about how important protein is, it's important to choose the best protein, which is a complete protein. Or, at the very least, you should make sure you are consuming foods that contain various essential amino acids, even if they don't have all of them. Below is a list of the nine essential amino acids, what they help the body with, and what foods you can find them in. As you can see, complete proteins are important for many reasons.

Amino Acid	Function	Foods
Histidine	Essential for healthy tissue repair and nervous system function.	beef, poultry, dairy, rice, wheat, rye, seafood, beans, cauliflower, mushrooms, potatoes, bamboo shoots, eggs, buckwheat, corn, bananas, cantaloupe, and citrus fruits
Valine	Important for muscle metabolism, tissue repair, nitrogen balance, and it can be used as an energy source by muscle tissue	cottage cheese, fish, poultry, sesame seeds, lentils, tofu, egg whites, peanuts, beef, lamb, and gelatin
Isoleucine	Essential for blood-clotting, blood sugar regulation, muscle repair, and transporting oxygen to the lungs	eggs, chicken, fish, cheese, soybeans, seaweed, turkey
Leucine	Important for energy, regulating glucose, and dissolving visceral fat	soybeans, beef, chicken, parmesan cheese, pork, seeds, nuts, and white beans
Phenylalanine	Essential for mood, skin pigment, and energy.	beef, poultry, pork, fish, milk, yogurt, eggs, cheese, soy, walnuts, and sunflower seeds
Threonine	Necessary for immune function, mood, wound healing, and the formation of bones, cartilage, hair, teeth,	cottage cheese, milk, eggs, sesame seeds, beans, poultry, fish, beef, lentils, and corn

	and nails, skeletal muscles, and the small intestines.	
Tryptophan	Important for appetite regulation, quality sleep, and the production of vitamin B3 (niacin) and serotonin	milk, chocolate, oats, bananas, dried dates, cottage cheese, turkey, peanuts
Methionine	Essential for metabolism and fighting oxidative stress	chicken, fish, milk, beef, eggs, nuts, grains, beans
Lysine	Important in the production of hormones, enzymes, and collagen (needed for bone, muscle, cartilage, and skin formation)	beef, fish, eggs, soy, poultry, nuts, and dairy

BCAAs and Thermogenesis

Of these nine essential amino acids listed above, three of them stand out even further: leucine, isoleucine, and valine. These are known as branched-chain amino acids or BCAAs. BCAAs are essential because they stimulate muscle protein synthesis, aka muscle growth, and prevent muscle wasting or muscle breakdown.

Why is muscle mass significant? Because when you increase muscle mass, you boost your resting metabolism, and that makes your body burn more calories which is especially helpful for people trying to lose weight.

In other words, eating protein looks like this:

- Eat protein > build muscle > burn more calories while resting

Burning calories brings me to another significant point regarding protein. Your body will "heat up" when you eat protein (this is known as the thermic effect). This happens because the body works harder to digest protein. (This explains why some people experience "the meat sweats" when eating high amounts of meat.) The body uses more energy to digest protein than it uses to digest other macronutrients. In fact, it's possible to burn 30 percent of your protein calories just while digesting them (that is if the protein comes from _lean_ protein foods).

In other words, eating protein also looks like this:

- Eat protein > create heat > burn calories during digestion

From these two bullet points, we see that eating protein (especially from BCAAs) causes the body to burn more calories both while resting and eating. Therefore protein should play an essential part in any weight loss strategy.

That being said, do not begin taking a high-dose BCAA supplement or dramatically increase your dietary intake without first consulting your doctor. Research has found that a high-sugar or a high-fat diet with BCAAs induced anxiety-like behavior in rats, which was not reversed with a selective serotonin reuptake inhibitor. (5)

Plant Protein Versus Animal Protein

As you see various meats, as well as eggs and dairy, are listed as "complete" proteins, and good sources of various essential amino acids. Again, these amino acids are "essential" because we cannot make them on our own, so it is "essential" that we consume them through diet. This is often very hard (but not impossible) for vegans because they do not eat many of the foods on this list.

There's a lot of disagreement out there whether animal or plant-based proteins are better for you. On one side, there is the argument that humans are better able to digest animal proteins because they are closer to our biological makeup, and they contain ALL the amino acids we need to live. On the other side, many say that plant-based proteins are easier to digest, healthier for you, and animal-based proteins are not necessary.

Again, as I said in the introduction of this book, to say that _one_ way is best for _all_ people is entirely erroneous. Humans are too unique to lump them all into one diet. So, I'm not going to choose a side here. My opinion is that both sides are correct, and both sides have issues. That's why it is crucial to take into consideration each person's unique make-up, genetic history, current health situation, location, and even shopping habits.

So, let's go over it all. First I'd like to talk about the downfalls to both.

One big downfall to consuming only plant-based protein is its incompleteness, BUT…. if you are diligent and calculated with your choices, you can certainly get around that by including complete plant proteins like quinoa, buckwheat, hemp, chia seeds, and spirulina. The other difficulty with only consuming plant proteins is that some of these (like quinoa and buckwheat) are more carb-heavy than meat, so they don't work well with a ketogenic diet and can sometimes pose problems for people with specific metabolic issues.

Also, some people who have (or are at risk for) certain autoimmune diseases, often have a difficult time with quinoa and buckwheat (as well as other grains and pseudo-grains). Another issue is that lectins (plant proteins) in these grains can cause inflammation and even damage to the gut lining (among other things) in people with autoimmune issues. Also, most grains contain a lectin similar in structure to gluten, so the body can experience what's called cross-reactivity. This means it reacts to the non-gluten grain as if it really was gluten simply because it resembles gluten. So, plant proteins that come from grains are definitely not for everyone.

Other things to consider are tastebuds and needs. Take me, for example. I have attention deficit issues and, in the past, have struggled a lot with anxiety and depression. Because of these two things, I need a lot of the amino acid tyrosine. I can get this from eating cauliflower, broccoli, avocados, and beets (which I absolutely love), but even if I ate huge portions of these every single day, it would still not meet my unique, personal needs. So a vegan diet would not work for me. I could also eat more dairy and eggs to get more tyrosine, but I do not feel very good eating those. So a vegetarian diet wouldn't work for me either. I personally feel best eating high amounts of protein (sometimes from chicken but mostly from fatty fish like salmon). This is in addition to my high-tyrosine veggies, of course. That's my "sweet spot," where my temple operates at its best—even though many of my close friends swear by the vegan diet. Again, it's all about finding what works for _you_.

Lastly, it is important to consider location. Some people simply do not have access to organic or non-GMO options at their local grocery store. So, in that case, it is definitely NOT better to eat plant proteins if they are genetically modified, especially when it comes to soy. In fact, there are many other downfalls to soy, too, which I will cover later in this book.

Animal Proteins

Animal proteins _do_ have a better absorption rate and availability to the body, and they _do_ contain many of the complete proteins. However, there can be downfalls to this, also. First, animal protein is often higher in sulfur-containing amino acids. This means that it can increase the acidity of the body, and possibly lead to calcium depletion when the body tries to balance out its pH level. (I will talk a lot more about pH in a later phase.) For now, though, just know that it can be an issue—though it is not typical if the meat is consumed in moderation with a well-balanced diet.

The other downfall to animal protein is how the animals are raised. Not all meat is the same. Organic, cage-free, free-range chicken is the only kind of chicken I recommend buying. Commercial non-organic chicken can be full of harmful bacteria. The chickens are also sometimes given hormones and antibiotics that can negatively affect the humans who consume the meat. This can contribute to gut issues, antibiotic resistance, and hormone imbalances, among other things. (I will talk more about this in later chapters also.) Animal studies even suggest that commercial chicken meat may be a cause of the development of PCOS (polycystic ovary syndrome). (6)

The same is often true when choosing beef. I only recommend eating organic, grass-fed beef. Non-organic animals that are not fed grass are fed grains. These can make their intestinal tracts much more acidic, which can promote the growth of harmful bacteria like E. coli. Cows that are not labeled organic are typically given antibiotics to prevent disease. In fact, 80% of antibiotics sold in the U.S. goes to livestock. (7) These animals are also often given hormones like estrogen to increase their weight (yielding more meat).

That being said, organic, grass-fed beef is one of the best proteins around, in my opinion. It is higher in omega 3s, vitamin E, antioxidants, and CLA (conjugated linoleic acid), which is believed to prevent cancer. (8) And according to an October 1999 article in the "Journal of Dairy Science," the CLA content in grass-fed cows is five times higher than that from grain-fed cows.

So, as you can see, both plant and animal proteins have their pros and cons. Neither one is "bad," but there are "bad versions" of both that are available at the supermarket. It's important to know the difference and choose the better option for you personally.

It's also important to remember that your choice may not be everyone else's choice. Some people simply don't like the taste of meat or don't like how animals are treated, so they choose to get their protein from plant sources. Some people can't do grains because of autoimmune issues, or some live in areas where non-GMO options just aren't available, so they have to rely on animal sources. Each unique person has a unique situation, lifestyle, taste preference, and belief system. Therefore, it's enormously unfair to assume there is only one "right" way to get protein. Please try to remember that. I see too many people "preaching protein" in all the wrong ways.

Other "Bad" Proteins

As I mentioned, genetically modified plant proteins, non-organic beef and poultry, and farm-raised seafood are on my list of bad proteins—not because the amino acids themselves are bad, but because there are other factors regarding the meat that far outweigh the benefits, in my opinion.

There is another type of protein that is also on my "bad" list—meat substitutes like Quorn, produced in the UK. Quorn is what's known as mycoprotein. It is formed by fermenting and processing a fungus called Fusarium venenatum found in soil. The problem is Fusarium venenatum is mold! Quorn is also processed. It's mixed in large vats with glucose, fixed nitrogen, synthetic vitamins, and minerals and then it's heat-treated at high temperatures.

Even though it is often touted as a plant-based, vegetarian protein, it is a long way from what I consider to be healthy food. Aside from being unsafe for people with mold allergies or mold sensitivities, it can also be harmful to gut health. Because of gut imbalances, many people do not have enough good bacteria in the gut to combat this fungus. This can then result in a fungal overgrowth because fungi are often more vicious and destructive than bacterial cultures. (I will talk much more about this in the next phase.)

Protein Shakes

As a health coach, I think one of the things I am asked about the most is protein powders and shakes. My clients take pictures of labels and send them to me to make sure they're healthy. *"Is this one ok?"* they ask. I'm not exaggerating when I say I've probably looked at 100 labels or more. And I'm so happy to do it because there are a lot—and I mean A LOT—of poorly made products on the market these days. And I do not want my clients to sabotage their health with unhealthy ingredients.

So, I'd like to give you a list of some of what I consider to be the worst ingredients found in various protein powders/shakes. As you know, I'm a big fan of getting protein from real food, but if you can't get enough from food because of allergies or busyness, or maybe you need a quick pre or post-workout snack, then yes, I'm a big fan of supplementing because protein is _that_ important.

However, when shopping, you have to read labels carefully. Even though protein is essential, a product with 25 grams of protein isn't doing you any good if it has a bunch of bogus ingredients in it that are ruining your gut health, causing inflammation, disrupting your blood sugars, and filling you with toxins. So, here are my own personal "No-Nos" that I stay clear of:

- Refined vegetable oils – things like canola, sunflower, soybean, safflower, or corn oil that are hydrogenated and cause inflammation. We've already talked a lot about why these are unhealthy, but it's important to know they are often added to protein powders and shakes because they're cheap to produce.
- Shelf stabilizers – Be on the lookout for things like carrageenan. Some researchers link carrageenan to things like suppressed immune function, ulcerative colitis, even colorectal cancer. In fact, it has been

demonstrated that when guinea pigs are supplied with degraded carrageenan in their drinking water, ulcerations develop in 100% of the animals in their large intestine by the end of 30 days. (9)

- Artificial Sweeteners – Things like sucralose, aspartame, Acesulfame K, Saccharin, and high fructose corn syrup, corn syrup, and corn syrup solids. If you see any of these listed on the label, PUT IT BACK! I will talk more about my reasoning on this in the next phase.

- Soy proteins – Some soy proteins come from genetically-modified sources and contain chemical compounds that can cause hormonal disturbances. (I will talk more about this in later chapters also.)

- Casein – While casein is not in itself bad for you (natural casein does have several health benefits), casein protein powder is often made in a lab using high heat or acid to extract the protein from the dairy. Therefore, it can contain toxic residues. What's more, heating casein at hot temperatures destroys certain amino acids in it. This "denatures" the protein, so it cannot be fully absorbed by the body. By the time it reaches the colon (undigested), it can start to ferment and produce ammonia. Casein also contains an opioid peptide that acts on opioid receptors in the body (the same opioid receptors that heroin and morphine act on.) This is why some people claim they have an "addiction to dairy," and can't give it up. The peptide can also cause inflammation in the GI tract and can kill healthy gut flora. (I will talk more about this in later chapters too.)

- Skim milk powders and milk solids – These ingredients are basically used to add "bulk" to cheap powders. So, when you see these listed, it should serve as a red flag that the protein powder is not of the highest quality. Powdered milk goes through many processes. In addition to being pasteurized, it is also usually filtered, evaporated, separated, and standardized, until at last it is heated at a high temperature and dried into a powder. Again, this is denatured and therefore, not digested well.

I know, the above list might sound daunting, especially if you love making protein shakes. I get it. I LOVE shakes, too. But don't worry. You don't have to give them up just because there are so many low-quality products on the market. They're not ALL bad. In fact, I personally use the Plexus Lean™ protein powders (in Chocolate, Vanilla, and Mocha), which are some of the highest-quality protein powders I've ever seen. Plexus Lean™ has ingredients I feel confident about. For example, the Plexus Lean™ Whey (chocolate and vanilla flavors) contain the following:

- 24 g of protein when prepared as directed, which includes a _complete_ amino acid profile, including BCAAs like leucine, isoleucine, and valine (but not a high-dose free form of BCAAS, like some other supplements)

- 5 g of fiber, including prebiotic fiber to support digestive health (I'll talk more about the importance of this in later chapters.)
- bioavailable forms of 24 vitamins and minerals
- highly bioavailable methylated folate (5-MTHF)
- digestive enzymes to aid in the digestion of whey protein
- lecithin, a source of choline, to support brain health
- Vitamin C to help fight free radical damage and help support a healthy immune system

What's important to note is that Plexus Lean contains an *rBGH-Free* whey protein. rBGH stands for recombinant bovine growth hormone, which is a hormone made in a lab using genetic technology. It is a synthetic version of the bovine somatotropin (BST), which is naturally produced in cows' pituitary glands. Monsanto developed this synthetic version from genetically engineered E. coli bacteria. (9) Today it is often injected into cows in order to boost milk production.

However, when cows are injected with rBGH, their levels of IGF-1 increase up to 20-fold. (9) IGF-1 is a hormone that acts on the pituitary gland that affects many things in the metabolic system. This IGF-1 is excreted in the cow's milk, and over the last three decades, about 50 scientific publications have documented that increased IGF-1 levels in hormone-treated milk increase your risk for breast, colon, and prostate cancers. (10)

This is one of the many reasons I choose Plexus. Because "rBGH-free whey" means the protein in Plexus Lean™ comes from animals that did not receive these hormones. What's more, whey protein is more thermogenic than any other protein, and has a host of other benefits:

- Whey protein increases total liver glutathione levels, which is a potent antioxidant (11)
- Whey protein promotes fat loss by enhancing the release of glucagon (builds muscle, burns fat) (12)
- Whey protein can boost energy expenditure by 80 to 100 calories per day and help people eat up to 441 fewer calories per day. One study showed that by eating 25% of daily calories in protein, it cut cravings by 60% and reduced late-night snacking by half. (13)

Lean Whey is also sweetened with a healthy, coconut palm sugar which ranks very well on the GI index. But I think the thing I love the most about Plexus Lean™ Whey is the taste. I consider myself to be somewhat of a "protein connoisseur," as I have tried many (and I mean MANY) brands and flavors over the years. Often, protein powders give me a chalky aftertaste. Lean does not, and is quite frankly the best-tasting protein powder I've tried, hands down. (For a list of Plexus Lean™ recipes, see the *Rebuilding Your Temple Workbook*.)

If you need a non-GMO, dairy-free option (also free of soy and gluten), you may want to consider Plexus Lean™ Vegetarian in Chocolate Mocha flavor. The following are what I consider to be its top-selling points:

- 20 grams of ultra-pure, plant-based, non-GMO protein from pea, rice, and six ancient grains (sacha inchi, amaranth, quinoa, buckwheat, millet, chia)
- Seven grams of dietary fiber, including prebiotic fiber like Fructooligosaccharides (FOS), Alpha-galactooligosaccharides (GOS), Xylooligosaccharides (XOS) to aid digestion and feed the good bacteria in the gut. (I'll talk more about this in the next phase.)
- Two grams of leucine for muscle support per serving (which has a much greater power to stimulate protein synthesis than any other amino acid.)
- Bacillus subtilis to help produce enzymes like amylase, protease, pullulanase, chitinase, xylanase, and lipase
- Ananas comosus which is beneficial for reproductive health, digestion and hunger control
- Highly bioactive 5-MTHF Folate that we talked about in the last chapter.
- Highly bioavailable and bioactive forms of other vitamins like B-Vitamins, Calcium, Vitamins A, D, and Zinc, among others
- Alpha-Linolenic Acid (ALA), a plant-based Omega-3 fatty acid that I mentioned at the beginning of Phase 2.

All forms of Plexus Lean™ are free of artificial flavors, artificial colors, artificial sweeteners, preservatives, cholesterol, carrageenan, and magnesium stearate. But even that's not the best part. For every serving of Plexus Lean you purchase (there are 14 servings in each package), Plexus®, through its philanthropic organization Plexus Charities, gives a contribution to Feeding America®—the nation's largest organization dedicated to fighting domestic hunger through a network of food banks. So you're getting healthy and helping to feed others who need nourishing as well. That's a win-win, in my opinion. I don't know of another protein that allows you to do that.

References:

(1) https://www.sciencedaily.com/releases/2014/01/140128202101.htm
(2) https://www.ncbi.nlm.nih.gov/pmc/articles/PMC5793233/
(3) https://www.ncbi.nlm.nih.gov/pubmed/20472480
(4) https://www.ncbi.nlm.nih.gov/pubmed/16469977
(5) https://www.ncbi.nlm.nih.gov/pubmed/23249694

(6) https://www.ncbi.nlm.nih.gov/pubmed/28625952
(7) https://www.marketwatch.com/story/80-of-antibiotics-sold-in-america-arent-used-to-treat-people-2015-04-29
(8) https://www.ncbi.nlm.nih.gov/pubmed/15941017
(9) https://www.ncbi.nlm.nih.gov/pmc/articles/PMC5410598/
(10) https://www.ncbi.nlm.nih.gov/pmc/articles/PMC3096574/
(11) https://articles.mercola.com/sites/articles/archive/2011/10/23/rgbh-in-milk-increases-risk-of-breast-cancer.aspx
(12) https://www.ncbi.nlm.nih.gov/pmc/articles/PMC4258944/
(13) https://www.healthline.com/nutrition/how-much-protein-per-day#what-it-is

Phase 4:

Rebuilding the Foundation

Materials: Fermented Foods, Raw Fruits and Vegetables

Tools: Plexus Slim®, Plexus® ProBio 5, Plexus xFactor Plus™, and Plexus VitalBiome™

Chapter 8: The City of the Microbiome

It is now time to begin Phase 4, where we will focus on one of the most important topics of any rebuild—THE FOUNDATION! If the foundation of a house isn't sturdy, the house itself isn't sturdy, regardless of how good the furnace, wiring, or framework is. And I believe it's the same with the temple of the body. If the foundation of the body isn't sturdy (aka healthy), then the body itself isn't completely healthy. It doesn't matter how much protein you eat or how many omegas you take. Plain and simple. So, the question then becomes: what is this the foundation of the temple of the body?

Well, Hippocrates summed it up perfectly when he said, "All disease begins in the gut." If all disease begins in the gut, then—on the flip side—that means true and lasting health begins in the gut also. So, the "foundation" then is GUT HEALTH, specifically the microbiome.

What is the microbiome? Well, the microbiome is like an ecosystem of bacteria, fungi, and yeasts that live inside of you and on your skin. It's a network of really tiny living microorganisms located in the gut, mouth, throat, skin, colon, and genital tract. And while the bacteria themselves are tiny, the microbiome as a whole is NOT tiny. Not even close.

The microbiome is made up of approximately 100 trillion microbial cells, as well as all of their genes. So, this is an enormous ecosystem! In fact, these bacterial cells outnumber our human cells 10 to 1. That means we are actually more "bug" than we are human!

But why are these little "buggers" so important? Why am I calling this topic the "foundation" of human health? Because the microbiome houses both good _and_ bad bacteria. (As you can imagine, it's important that the good guys outnumber the bad guys.)

What's more, there are different types or "strains" of bacteria in the microbiome. Think of it like a forest that houses different types of animals. There's not just one type of animal living in a forest (like just squirrels), and there's not just one single animal from each of the animal types (one squirrel, one deer, etc.). There are many of each type! Such is the case with the microbiome, too. There are many microorganisms of many types.

Microbial Jobs

While the microbiome houses many living organisms from many different strains, what makes it so very important to overall health is the fact that each of these strains has one or more jobs to do inside the body. Like a community of individuals who work together to keep things running smoothly, so these microbes work together (and independently) to keep the body healthy.

So, what are some of these "jobs" that microbes have? Well, they supply important vitamins to the body. They fight pathogens, harmful bacteria, viruses, and diseases. They make up about 70 percent of the immune system. They affect the way we store fat, how we balance blood sugar, how fast or slow our metabolism is. They help control how our genes express themselves. Some of these bacteria even regulate the body's response to inflammation.

What's more, the microbiome is also very closely connected to the brain. In fact, embedded in the wall of the gut, there is what's known as the enteric nervous system (or ENS). The ENS works by itself like a second brain, and it works in conjunction with the brain in your head, too. That's where the term "gut instinct" comes from, or the phrase "nervous stomach," or "butterflies in your stomach." These terms come from your gut-brain...which, even though it's dubbed a "second" brain, does not mean it's a *small* brain.

Your ENS has approximately 500 million neurons, which is more than the spine! The ENS doesn't make important decisions like your "head brain," but it does communicate with it. How? It talks to the brain along a pathway called the Vagus Nerve (as well as other systems). Think of it like a telephone landline where two people talk back and forth. (*"Head Brain? Hello, this is Gut Brain."*)

Because of this two-way communication between the two brains, it's easy to see why studies are now showing that mental health impacts gut health, and gut health impacts mental health. Studies even show that poor gut health can lead to neurological and neuropsychiatric disorders. (1) (2)

Research also shows that gut microbes influence the brain's hypothalamic-pituitary-adrenal axis. (3) (What the heck is that? It's another "highway of communication," this one involved in the stress response, among other things. I will talk more about stress in later chapters.)

If that wasn't enough, gut microbes produce 30 different neurotransmitters, they secrete hormones, and they regulate the expression of hormones. Think of it this way: the microbiome acts as a sort of master control center for hormone balance. I suppose this is why experts now consider the microbiome a "virtual endocrine gland." (3)

Now, what are some of the hormones and neurotransmitters that are produced in the gut by the microbiome? Well, for starters, 90% of serotonin is produced in the gut. This is what influences a happy mood, helps regulate appetite, and serves as a precursor for melatonin, helping you sleep. In fact, the gut-brain connection itself is dependent on serotonin.

The gut also produces dopamine, which plays a role in focus, attention, learning, motivation, and reward (as I mentioned in earlier chapters). It is also a key player in addiction.

There is also an estrogen-gut connection, too. There is a group of bacteria in the gut called the estrobolome, which is responsible for breaking excess estrogen so that there is not too much of it. What's more, estrogen is made by the ovaries. It circulates through the body to where it's needed, then the liver deactivates it, and it is flushed out of the body through the bowels.

However, certain bad bacteria can produce an enzyme called beta-glucuronidase, that can re-activate estrogen in the gut causing it to reenter the bloodstream. This combined with a weakened estrobolome (which is supposed to remove excess estrogen) can result in hormone imbalances that often play a role in infertility, PMS, heavy bleeding, cramps, and PCOS.

The gut also produces norepinephrine which is a hormone that triggers the "fight or flight" response in stressful situations. (4) In fact, some of the bacteria that produce high levels of this stress hormone are infective bacteria like e. Coli and salmonella. Even thyroid hormones are connected to the gut because specific gut bacteria help convert about 20% of the inactive thyroid hormone T4 into the active form T3.

So, why do I consider gut health (specifically the microbiome) to be the FOUNDATION of the temple of the body? Because of all these super important things that I just mentioned. It will be very difficult to get healthy if you do not take care of your microbiome. Plain and simple.

Microbial Wreck-It-Ralphs

Now that we've gone over the jobs of some of the "good guys" living in the microbiome let's talk about a strain of "bad guys." There is a type of yeast living in the microbiome called Candida Albicans. (There are actually many kinds of Candida, but Candida Albicans is the most common.) Technically, Candida is both good and bad, and everyone has it. We acquire it from our mother in the birth canal the day we enter the world. We are supposed to have it because it, too, has a job to do. It assists in digestion and nutrient absorption to a degree. But its main job is to decompose the body when we die.

Yuck, I know. But here's how it works: Candida feeds on byproducts and dead cells in the body. When we die, they feed generously, then multiply and "come into their own," I guess you could say. The once-harmless yeast then morphs into a very destructive and pathogenic organism. Candida grows tentacles so that it can burrow down into its host, and it shoots threads of itself throughout tissue for a quicker and more invasive takeover of the body.

Usually, Candida is harmless to us because it is kept at bay by the immune system—that is until it gets the "go ahead" at death when the immune system shuts off. The problem is, byproducts and dead cells are not the only things Candida feed on. It also feeds on sugar. So, those who eat a high carb/high sugar diet can experience a Candida overgrowth while they are still living.

This can become a MAJOR problem because Candida is so destructive by nature. Candida is like the town demolition crew or a strain of Wreck-It Ralphs in the city of the microbiome. When it grows and multiplies and morphs with its tentacles, it's going to try to do its job. It's going to try to decompose the body, even though the body isn't dead yet.

Because it lives in the microbiome, it starts demolition where it's at: in the gut. The intestinal lining is built like a concrete block foundation under a house. Blocks are held together by mortar. Likewise, the cells of the gut lining are held together by connecting junctions known as "tight junction proteins." These junctions are porous enough to let important nutrients and fluid pass into the body, but tight enough to prevent larger things like toxins and bacteria from passing through.

When Candida burrows into the intestinal lining, it creates holes in these junctions. This situation has become known as Leaky Gut Syndrome. Why is this a problem? One, because now Candida has an open door to the rest of the body. This makes it easier for it to run rampant and do its dirty work on other tissue and organs.

Two, when the gut is "leaky," partially digested food proteins and fats can slip out into the bloodstream. When this happens, the immune system can send out a red flag that there is a foreign substance present. (It's not that the food itself is foreign to the body, but that it is foreign to that particular AREA of the body. Food isn't supposed to be in the blood.) Once the body sends out this red flag, it will "remember" it, so that that the next time the food enters the body, the immune response is triggered more quickly and easily. This is how a food allergy can develop.

What's more, when leaky gut continues for an extended time, more and more things slip out into the bloodstream, like toxins, bacteria, viruses, and byproducts. The immune system increases inflammation and works overtime to try and combat all this. Unfortunately, the immune system is not very good under pressure like that. It goes haywire and can even start to misfire because of something called molecular mimicry, which I talked about at the beginning of this book. But it's important enough to go over again. Molecular mimicry is where the substances that leak from the gut, "mimic" or look like the body's own cells. So, the immune system, thinking it's the foreign invader, attacks its own tissue instead. This is how autoimmune disease develops.

When the immune system attacks the thyroid, it's called Hashimoto's or Grave's disease; when it attacks the small intestine it's called Celiac disease; when it attacks the protective covering of nerves it's called Multiple Sclerosis, and so forth and so on. This is such a widespread problem that there are now more than 80 diseases that are classified as having an autoimmune nature to them. EIGHTY!!

Now, Candida Albicans is not the one and only culprit for Leaky Gut Syndrome. (Other things like toxins, medications, etc. can wear away those junctions too, which I will talk about later.) But Candida is among the most common culprits because of the standard American diet, which is so full of sugar and carbs.

Killing Candida

Clearly, if you have an overgrowth of Candida, it is essential to talk to your doctor about getting rid of that immediately. An excellent first step is to stop eating sugar and to stop carb-loading, which you accomplish through a ketogenic diet. The elimination of carbs and sugar can help starve the yeast by removing their food source from the body. Unfortunately, though, that is not always enough, especially if you have an accumulation of other things like byproducts and dead cells that they can use. You also need to "actively" attack them, too, which is not as easy as you might think.

Many people will say you need to start taking probiotics to combat Candida, and that is half true. When you take probiotics, you are recruiting more good guys into the battle, which helps "balance the sides" so to speak and resolve dysbiosis (imbalance). However, Candida albicans have very impressive armor. They have a sturdy cell wall that surrounds them, sort of like a full-body, bullet-proof vest. Approximately 80 to 90% of this cell wall is made of carbohydrates such as glucan and chitin, as well as some proteins such as fibrin and a few fats. (5) (Another reason why it's crucial to limit carbohydrates.)

This cell wall not only gives shape to the yeast and helps it morph and adapt to the changing environment of the body, but it is also essential to the life and work of the yeast. The cell wall has specific "grips" that enable Candida to stick to cells and other materials in the body. (Think Velcro.) This ability to "stick" is what promotes widespread infection.

Not only that, it is well documented that the cell wall components (glucan, chitin, and mannoproteins) can activate or depress immune responses. (5) In fact, some components in the cell wall can control the action of nearly all arms of the immune system (natural killer cells, phagocytic cells, cell-mediated immunity, and humoral mechanisms). I hope you are starting to see how big of a deal this is.

If that wasn't bad enough, Candida can also form biofilms. Essentially, the yeasts ban together to create an organized community (like an army), then attach as a group to a surface in the body and hide in an environment of material (like a bunker). These biofilms can be anywhere from 25 to 450 micrometers (μm) thick and can appear within the first 24 hours after they settle into the host.

It's also important to note that Candida biofilms are made up of about 32% glucose. (6) That means Candida not only needs sugar to live and reproduce, but they also need it to make a biofilm where they can hide from the immune system. This is another reason why the low-carb, no-sugar ketogenic diet is often beneficial.

What also makes the biofilm so problematic is the old saying, "power in numbers." When Candida yeasts ban together, they behave differently than they do on their own. They get "cocky," and are very resistant to treatment. Typically, antifungals such as fluconazole, nystatin, amphotericin B, and chlorhexidine are prescribed to combat yeast overgrowth, but studies show biofilms make Candida cells highly resistant to these medications. (7) One study actually showed "a near-TOTAL resistance to antifungal agents by biofilm-associated Candida." (8)

So, my point is: just "crowding out" Candida with typical probiotics is often NOT enough. To eradicate this organism, it's crucial to focus on the biofilm and the cell wall. You need to remove their armor and destroy their bunker with very specific tools. The tool I believe is most effective for this is task is Plexus® ProBio 5.

Here's why: at the time of manufacture, each capsule of ProBio 5 not only has 2 billion colony-forming units (CFU) of "good guys" from five different strains, it also contains four critical enzymes that I consider to be the secret weapons. These are Serrapeptase, Proteases, Chitosanase, Cellulase.

Why are these important? First, because Candida are not resistant to enzymes and cannot create resistance to them like they can with some antifungal medications. Second, these particular enzymes are capable of breaking down the materials present in the Candida structure. For example:

- Serrapeptase is a type of enzyme that helps breakdown the fibrin in the cell wall of Candida. This is crucial because the fibrin layer is what allows Candida "stick" to its host. So, if fibrin is broken down, the yeast cannot attach to human cells. (9)
- Protease is a type of enzyme that not only helps break down the proteins in the cell wall of Candida, but also the protein in its nucleus.
- Chitosanase is an enzyme that helps break down chitin. Chitin is a fibrous substance (deriving from glucose), that is the main component of the exoskeleton or the hard, outer shell of Candida.
- Cellulase is an enzyme that helps breakdown cellulose, which is one of the components that make up Candida biofilm. These biofilms are also made of fibrinogen and fibronectin, so they are also vulnerable to the enzyme Serrapeptase listed above.
- ProBio 5 also has 250% of the DV of Vitamin C and 125% of the DV of Vitamin B6, which are both valuable for immune support. Additionally, it has 25 mg of grape seed extract, which is a powerful antioxidant that not only supports the immune system but is also very effective against Candida. In fact, studies show that grape seed extract alone can inhibit the growth of Candida yeast cells. (10)

I hope you are starting to understand the severity of this. Candida should not be taken lightly, given how destructive and insidious it is. So please, take this information to heart and discuss ProBio 5 with your doctor. I consider this to be the single, most-effective tool you can use when combatting Candida and rebuilding the temple foundation.

That being said, coconut oil also has many benefits. As I mentioned earlier, coconut oil is made up of three different medium-chain fatty acids – caprylic acid, capric acid, and lauric acid. Caprylic acid has strong antifungal properties, specifically helpful against Candida. In fact, one study showed that mice fed coconut oil had a 10-fold drop in the colonization of Candida Albicans yeast in their gut. (11) What makes caprylic acid so effective is its ability to puncture the cell wall, which causes the yeast to rupture. (12) This is another benefit to adopting a ketogenic diet that includes fat bombs and other foods made with coconut oil. (Recipes can be found in the *Rebuilding Your Temple Workbook*.)

How Can You Tell if You Have Candida?

At this point, you may be concerned about the possibility of having a Candida overgrowth. As I mentioned, a diet high in sugar and carbs can increase the risk because Candida feeds on sugar. But there are other things that can increase the risk also. Below is a list of questions regarding other possible contributors. If you can answer yes to more than a few of these, it may be worth discussing the possibility with your doctor.

Part 1: "Have You Ever....?"

(1) Have you ever taken antibiotics, steroids, or birth control pills?
(2) Have you ever had a soda habit of more than 2/week?
(3) Have you ever taken any OTC meds like ibuprofen, sleep aids or allergy meds, etc. regularly for over a week straight?
(4) Have you ever used Splenda, Equal or Sweet 'n Low more than twice/week?
(5) Have you ever had an alcohol habit of more than three drinks/week for two or more weeks/month?
(6) Have you ever been chronically sleep-deprived getting less than 7 hours of sleep/night for more than a week straight?
(7) Have you ever eaten poorly for an extended time, even as a child? (This includes items like cookies, candy, soft drinks, processed breakfast cereals, peanut butter and jelly sandwiches, boxed snack cakes, juice boxes, etc.)

Below is a list of questions regarding possible Candida symptoms. If you can answer yes to more than a few of these, it may be worth discussing these with your doctor also.

Part 2: "Do You Now...?"

(1) Do you feel like sugar or high carbohydrate foods sometimes control your life?
(2) Do you find it difficult to shake chronic health issues like skin rashes, sinus problems, or digestive problems even though you try to live a healthy life?
(3) Do you suffer reoccurring headaches or migraines?
(4) Do you get reoccurring vaginal yeast infections or instances of thrush?

(5) Do healthy foods like sauerkraut and kombucha cause negative symptoms or make you feel like you have a "buzz"?

(6) Do you get a stuffy nose or itchy after a glass of wine?

(7) Do you have issues such as chronic fatigue, brain fog, poor memory, exhaustion, insomnia, dizziness, or random aches and pains?

(8) Do you have reoccurring cystitis or urinary tract infections?

(9) Do you have abdominal issues such as bloating, flatulence, cramps, acid reflux, indigestion, and/or burping after meals?

(10) Do you have skin issues such as hives, acne, Rosacea, discolored nails, athlete's foot, tinea, or Psoriasis?

(11) Do you have mouth issues such as bad breath, cracked tongue, white tongue, or cracks in the corners of your mouth?

(12) Do you have respiratory issues such as chronic sinusitis, nasal congestion, postnasal drip, hay fever, or asthma?

(13) Do you have hormone issues such as PMS, irregular cycle, infertility, etc.?

(14) Do you have emotional issues such as anxiety, depression, panic attacks, irritability, or mood swings?

(15) Do you have ADD, ADHD or trouble focusing?

(16) Do you have weight issues such as weight gain, weight that won't come off, inflammation, and/or fluid retention?

(17) Do you have other, seemingly random, symptoms such as Tinnitus (ringing in the ears), sensitivity to smells such as chemicals and perfumes, or itchy ears, eyes or anus?

(18) Do you have cravings after dinner where you do not feel "complete" without something sweet to eat?

(19) Do you use acid-blocking medications or have an H. pylori infection?

If you and your doctor feel that there is a possibility of Candida, your practitioner may want to test you for it. This can be done by testing stool, urine, and/or blood samples. You can also perform an easy (though not 100% accurate) test at home.

Even though Candida resides in the intestines, it can sometimes travel along the mucous membranes of the digestive tract into the stomach, up the esophagus, into the mouth. If this happens, you can test for the presence of Candida by doing a simple saliva spit test first thing in the morning.

Place a glass of plain water next to your bed in the evening. As soon as you wake up, before you put anything into your mouth, work up a bunch of saliva in the mouth, and then spit it gently into the glass. After 3 minutes, inspect the glass.

- Saliva that is clear and floats on the top of the glass = no Candida

- Saliva that is floating, but has strings hanging down toward the bottom of the glass = Candida likely
- Saliva that is cloudy and sinks to the bottom of the glass = Candida likely
- Saliva that makes cloudy particles within the water = Candida likely

Again, this is not 100% accurate because, as I said, this is only detected in the water *if* the Candida has traveled to the mouth. Sometimes it does not but instead wreaks havoc on other parts of the body. It is best to talk to your doctor about these concerns.

Die-Off Symptoms

If you and your doctor detect the presence of Candida and you begin to eradicate it with ProBio 5 or antifungals, it's essential to go slow and stay in close contact with your practitioner.

When large numbers of candida cells are killed too quickly, it is possible to experience "die-off symptoms." As candida dies these organisms release into the body all of the nasty substances they contain—which includes 70 different toxins, like ethanol, uric acid, and acetaldehyde. Naturally, this can make you feel lousy.

Candida die-off symptoms vary from person to person, because each person has different degrees of overgrowth and likely different kinds of Candida. But symptoms are often compared to the common cold or seasonal allergies. The toxic byproducts of Candida can cause inflammation, which can lead to a stuffy nose, blocked sinuses, and other allergy-like symptoms. Acetaldehyde can also cause things like brain fog, fatigue, headaches, and nausea, even a sore abdomen (near the liver, especially).

These are some other possible symptoms of Candida die-off that should be discussed with your doctor:

- Nausea
- Headache, fatigue, dizziness
- Swollen glands
- Bloating, gas, constipation or diarrhea
- Increased joint or muscle pain
- Elevated heart rate
- Chills, cold feeling in your extremities
- Body itchiness, hives or rashes
- Sweating
- Fever
- Skin breakouts

- Recurring vaginal and/or sinus infections

If you have these or any die-off symptoms, you and your doctor, you may want to slow down your treatment. You may need to just go slower and ease into ProBio5 more gradually.

Also, your doctor may advise that you take additional vitamin C and a supplement like molybdenum or milk thistle to assist the liver as it is the main pathway for eliminating toxins. Die-Off symptoms can mean that that pathway is overwhelmed.

Some find it beneficial to increase their water intake to help these toxins out of the body. A sauna or steamy shower could also help expel toxins quicker.

While these symptoms can be uncomfortable, it's important not to get discouraged and quit the protocol. (Unless your doctor advises it—remember your doctor is the contractor on this rebuild!) Feeling bad is often a good sign that progress is being made—and besides, it doesn't last forever. Typically die-off lasts just a few days or a week… though some people have experienced issues for a few weeks, depending on the severity of the overgrowth. Again, it is absolutely essential to stay in contact with your doctor or healthcare provider as you go through this. Do not do this without the help of a professional.

Military Microbes, AKA "The Good Guys"

The Microbiome is supposed to be an environment where you have more good guys than bad guys. As I mentioned, there are strains of good bacteria that do many important things in the body like assist metabolism, and make hormones and neurotransmitters, etc. But there are also strains of good guys whose job it is to help combat the bad guys.

These beneficial microbes are in charge of stimulating the activation of immune cells. They're like military generals that tell the ground troops of your immune system what to do. They help your immune system's T cells develop, and they teach them the difference between a foreign invader and the body's own tissue. This is important in preventing autoimmune disease (or any illness, really).

More than 70 percent of your immune system is located in the gut. In fact, the intestines contain more immune cells than the whole rest of the body combined. So, this is kind of a big deal.

These microbes have an important job because the immune system needs to be working at its best at all times—not sluggish, but not too alert either. When the "generals" become scarce, the army of the immune system is compromised, and it can't respond the way it needs to. This gives the opposing forces (the bad, pathogenic bacteria) an upper hand—it gives them free rein in the microbial community.

This imbalance between good and bad bacteria is called gut dysbiosis, and it's incredibly harmful to overall health. When this happens, you can end up with a body that is not only struggling to perform its most basic functions for life but has become a sitting duck for infection and disease.

I hope by now, you are starting to see how important it is to protect the good guys. To do that, we first need to understand what causes them harm, so that we can avoid those things. So, let's go over them now.

Processed food

Anything boxed or canned can potentially disrupt gut flora depending on the amount and types of additives, chemicals, and preservatives added to the food. For example, emulsifiers which are additives that help oil and water blend (and are in many—and I mean MANY—processed foods) have been shown to alter the mucus barrier in the gut, (13) as well as the microbes associated with it. In fact, one study showed that mice fed the common emulsifiers carboxymethylcellulose and polysorbate-80 had an altered bacterial composition and thinner intestinal mucus, which led to weight gain, increased food consumption, increased fat mass, and impaired glucose handling. The mice also showed intestinal inflammation and metabolic syndrome. Some mice even developed colitis. (14) This is yet another reason why I just eat real food.

Artificial Sweeteners

Because artificial sweeteners pass through the GI tract without being digested, they can actually come in direct contact with bacteria in the colon. Studies on mice have shown that after this contact, over 40 different groups of bacteria were significantly altered in the microbiome—forty groups! (15) While I can't go over all forty of these groups, let's at least look at a few of them.

One of the groups of good bacteria affected by artificial sweeteners is lactobacilli. These microbes are important because they increase immune response, and they make lactic acid and other acids that prevent harmful bacteria from sticking to the body and multiplying. They're like soldiers in the microbial community.

Another group affected is bifidobacterial, which sticks to cells in the intestines, and help protect the lining from toxins and germs, so that they can't get into the blood. Another group significantly affected is Akkermansia. Ironically, Akkermansia controls metabolism. So, the little no-calorie artificial sweetener that is often pitched as a "healthy" no-sugar, diet sweetener, actually can kill the microorganisms that control your metabolism and cause weight gain. Ironic, isn't it?

Antibiotics

While antibiotics can be beneficial for killing or inhibiting various bacterial infections, it is important to remember that antibiotics aren't selective in their attack. What I mean is, they often don't just go after the bad guys. Antibiotics are anti-bacterial—in most cases, that means bad guys *and* good guys.

Studies have shown that antibiotics can affect about 30% of the bacteria in the gut, causing a swift decline not only in numbers of bacteria but also diversity of groups. (16) Once a person stops taking antibiotics, the microbiota can bounce back, yes— but often only to a degree. These antibiotic-induced changes in a person's microbiome can remain for long periods of time—months, even years. (17) Studies even now suggest that the microbiome may not ever bounce back to its original state! (18)

What's more, the remaining bacteria that are left after antibiotic exposure don't always operate in the same way. They can suffer from damaged cell membranes, which changes how they behave in the body. It affects gene expression, increases antibiotic resistance, and alters stress responses, among other things. (19)

These microbiome changes also increase the susceptibility of infection because antibiotics take out the generals and the soldiers. This leaves a person vulnerable to an overgrowth of harmful bacteria if they acquire it directly after taking antibiotics. Some of these can cause stubborn, long-term recurrent (even deadly) infections, like Clostridium Difficile. (20) (21)

GMOs

It's been estimated that more than 80% of genetically modified (GM) crops grown worldwide are engineered to tolerate being sprayed with glyphosate herbicides, the best-known being Roundup. (22) The benefit to farmers is that this herbicide kills all the nearby weeds but does not kill the crop. It sounds great for farmers, but what about those eating the produce laced with herbicides?

Unfortunately, glyphosate acts like an antimicrobial/antibacterial atomic bomb on the microbiome, wiping out good bacteria that help keep us free from disease. In fact, researchers have proposed that glyphosate is the most important causal factor in Celiac disease. (23) In fact, fish that are exposed to glyphosate develop digestive problems that are reminiscent of celiac disease. And, Celiac disease is commonly associated with imbalances in gut bacteria that can be adequately explained by the known effects of glyphosate on gut bacteria. (23)

While I believe processed food, artificial sweeteners, antibiotics, and GMOs are some of the most significant contributors to gut changes, they are not the only ones. Some other things that can be damaging to the microbiome are:

- Various over-the-counter products and medications: Things like mouthwashes, aspirin, antacids, painkillers, and laxatives can affect the microbiome. A recent 2018 study found that more than 800 products had antibacterial effects. In fact, 40 medications reduced the numbers of more than ten different strains of bacteria, and more than 25% of non-antibiotic drugs stalled the growth of at least one strain of gut bacteria. (24) And non-steroidal anti-inflammatory drugs (NSAIDs) like ibuprofen can cause a substantial increase in harmful bacteria in the gut. (25)
- Chlorinated drinking water: Chlorine kills all bacteria, regardless of whether they are good or bad. It may be beneficial to invest in a water purifier.
- Artificial food coloring: Most synthetic food dyes come from petroleum, or crude oil, and can contribute to intestinal inflammation potentially resulting in a leaky gut lining. This exposes the otherwise protected friendly flora and can allow harmful bacteria to spread throughout the body. What's more, food dyes can bind to proteins which the body cannot then break down (which is why children get colored lips when sucking lollipops). This, too, can cause inflammation from digestive distress. Additionally, researchers found that 73 percent of children with ADHD responded favorably to an elimination diet that included removing artificial colors. (26) Brain scans conducted by Amen Clinics also clearly demonstrates that Red Dye #40 can dramatically affect brain function. (27)
- Proton pump inhibitors (PPIs): PPIs have been found in animal studies to negatively alter the gut microbiome, with a significantly lower abundance and diversity of gut bacteria. (28) (29)

The Non-Ingestible Culprits

So far, I have mentioned several things that can be ingested that can harm the microbiome. But there are other, non-ingestible things that can wreak havoc on your gut too. Here are my top-two most commonly overlooked culprits:

Not enough sleep

A recent study conducted at Uppsala University in Sweden showed that a lack of sleep affects the microbiome. (30) Researchers followed nine healthy volunteers, who had regular sleeping habits before the study. The data collected showed that not getting enough sleep for just two consecutive nights affected the participants gut flora. It did not alter the diversity of strains very much, but the levels of each strain changed. They also found that the participants were 20% less receptive to insulin after two nights of sleep deprivation, and their gut flora resembled the gut flora of participants in other studies who were either clinically obese or had metabolic disorders.

What's more, research shows that the intestinal microbiome is regulated by circadian rhythms (the body's internal 24-hour clock, or its sleep-wake cycle) (31) and so, a disruption in this rhythm can impact the health and work of the microbiome. In fact, studies show that circadian disruption like jet lag can result in gut dysbiosis. (32)

While sleep clearly affects the microbiome, the microbiome also affects sleep. It's like "what came first, the chicken or the egg?" Certain bacteria in the gut assist in the transportation of serotonin, which helps regulate many functions in the body, including sleep, mood, and appetite. So not getting enough sleep could alter the gut to where, once you do want to sleep, you might not be able to. There begins the vicious cycle.

Stress

Animal studies conducted by scientists from Georgia State University in Atlanta found that a single exposure to social stress causes a change in the gut microbiota, similar to what is seen following other, much more severe physical stressors, and this change gets bigger following repeated exposures. (33)

Another study done by scientists from Ohio State University found that stress exposure led to changes in composition, diversity, and number of gut microorganisms. The bacterial communities not only became less diverse; they also had greater numbers of harmful bacteria like Clostridium. What's more, their data found that not only does stress change the bacteria levels in the gut, but that these changes can, in turn, impact immunity. (34)

How Do I Know?

At this point, you are probably beginning to see how important the city of the microbiome is, and why I refer to it as the foundation of the temple. This probably has made you curious as to what your "city" looks like and whether or not you have dysbiosis—more good guys than bad guys. Maybe you're asking yourself, "How do I know?"

This is a good question. After all, we are talking about microbes that are invisible to the naked eye, and ones that live inside us. We can't just take a look and see. Or can we?

As technology advances, this is becoming more and more possible. I encourage you to talk to your doctor about microbiome testing if you want to get an accurate picture of the microbes inside of you. You can also use online testing companies such as Viome.

Viome uses two pieces of technology: Metatranscriptomic Sequencing Technology & Artificial Intelligence. The metatranscriptomic sequencing technology has the power to see every microbial strain, the activity of these organisms, and whether they are producing nutrients or toxins inside the gut. The Viome artificial intelligence engine then runs multiple analyses to determine what foods and supplements are ideal for your unique gut microbiome.

It's a relatively simple process that I've used personally multiple times. You just order a testing kit online at www.Viome.com, when the test kit arrives you collect a stool sample, and then mail it back to Viome. While you wait for your results, you must register your kit online or in the app, using the kit ID number. You also must take a few online surveys regarding your current health. When Viome is finished processing your stool sample, your results will be posted in your online account with dietary recommendations.

This can be enormously helpful, especially when dealing with "mysterious GI issues." Take my daughter, for example. She struggled with intense stomach pains for more than a year. We removed dairy and wheat from her diet due to sensitivities. We eliminated all processed food. We saw several doctors who were able to rule out many diseases but, could not pinpoint the cause of her pain. Some began to speak in umbrella terms such as irritable bowel syndrome. Others suggested a diet of generally "safe foods" such as rice and chicken to rule out other possible food sensitivities, which we did. However, her symptoms did not change, and no causes could be determined.

My husband and I then ordered her a kit from Viome. Her results showed the presence of many pathogenic bacteria, fungi, and viruses and a low richness or diversity of strains. One of the most exciting findings was the presence of a virus known as Oryza sativa endornavirus—a plant virus associated with rice.

This was an important finding because we had removed wheat from her diet and replaced it with gluten-free options containing mostly rice. We also had been feeding her even more rice to rule out other sensitivities. While rice usually is "safe" for most people, it was not safe for our daughter because of the rice virus living in her microbiome. The more rice she ate, the more the virus ate (with the potential to grow and reproduce) and the more her pain increased.

Once again, what is good for one person isn't always good for everyone.

References:

(1) https://www.ncbi.nlm.nih.gov/pmc/articles/PMC5558112/
(2) https://www.ncbi.nlm.nih.gov/pmc/articles/PMC4662178/
(3) https://www.ncbi.nlm.nih.gov/pubmed/27345323
(4) https://www.sciencedirect.com/science/article/pii/S0925443904002182
(5) https://www.ncbi.nlm.nih.gov/pmc/articles/PMC98909/
(6) https://www.ncbi.nlm.nih.gov/pubmed/16849719
(7) https://www.ncbi.nlm.nih.gov/pmc/articles/PMC95423/?report=reader#!po=5.00 000
(8) https://www.ncbi.nlm.nih.gov/pmc/articles/PMC127206/
(9) https://pdfs.semanticscholar.org/1a18/b5c740bf9b403241c2176308ea058975740 1.pdf
(10) https://www.ncbi.nlm.nih.gov/pubmed/17913484
(11) http://msphere.asm.org/content/1/1/e00020-15
(12) https://www.ncbi.nlm.nih.gov/pubmed?cmd=Retrieve&db=PubMed&list_uids=11 600381&dopt=AbstractPlus
(13) https://www.ncbi.nlm.nih.gov/pubmed/29968743
(14) https://www.nih.gov/news-events/nih-research-matters/food-additives-alter-gut-microbes-cause-diseases-mice
(15) https://chriskresser.com/how-artificial-sweeteners-wreak-havoc-on-your-gut/
(16) http://journals.plos.org/plosbiology/article?id=10.1371/journal.pbio.0060280
(17) https://www.ncbi.nlm.nih.gov/pubmed?Db=pubmed&Cmd=ShowDetailView&Ter mToSearch=18043614
(18) https://www.ncbi.nlm.nih.gov/pubmed?Db=pubmed&Cmd=ShowDetailView&Ter mToSearch=20847294
(19) https://www.ncbi.nlm.nih.gov/pubmed?Db=pubmed&Cmd=ShowDetailView&Ter mToSearch=18043614
(20) https://www.ncbi.nlm.nih.gov/pubmed?Db=pubmed&Cmd=ShowDetailView&Ter mToSearch=12763508
(21) https://www.ncbi.nlm.nih.gov/pubmed?Db=pubmed&Cmd=ShowDetailView&Ter mToSearch=18363274
(22) https://detoxproject.org/glyphosate/whats-the-connection-between-glyphosate-and-genetically-modified-crops/
(23) https://www.ncbi.nlm.nih.gov/pmc/articles/PMC3945755/
(24) https://www.nature.com/articles/nature25979
(25) https://www.ncbi.nlm.nih.gov/pubmed/26482265
(26) http://calmglow.com/pdfs/food-allergies-and-ADHD.pdf
(27) https://www.amenclinics.com/blog/brain-health-guide-red-dye-40/
(28) https://www.ncbi.nlm.nih.gov/pubmed/26657899

(29) https://www.ncbi.nlm.nih.gov/pubmed/26719299
(30) https://www.ncbi.nlm.nih.gov/pmc/articles/PMC5123208/
(31) https://www.ncbi.nlm.nih.gov/pubmed/27793218
(32) https://insights.ovid.com/pubmed?pmid=26628099
(33) https://www.sciencedirect.com/science/article/pii/S0166432817316650
(34) https://www.sciencedaily.com/releases/2011/03/110321094231.htm

Chapter 9: Tools and Tips for Digestion

Disclaimer: These statements have not been evaluated by the Food and Drug Administration. None of the information in this book is intended to diagnose, treat, cure, or prevent any disease. All information contained in this chapter and this book are for educational purposes only and are not intended to replace the advice of a medical doctor. Stacy Malesiewski is not a doctor and does not give medical advice, prescribe medication, or diagnose illness. Stacy is a certified health coach, journalist, and an independent Plexus ambassador. These are her personal beliefs and are not the beliefs of Plexus Worldwide, Gray Matter Media, Inc., or any other named professionals in this book. If you have a medical condition or health concern, it is advised that you see your physician immediately. It is also recommended that you consult your doctor before implementing any new health strategy or taking any new supplements. Results may vary.

In the last chapter, I discussed the microbiome and the many things that can do it harm. In this chapter, I would like to talk about the things that can do it good. Obviously, if you have a likelihood of dysbiosis (60% of Americans do), it is important to repopulate the microbiome with good guys. Talk to your doctor about doing this with quality microencapsulated probiotics, like Plexus® ProBio 5.

Probiotics are the good guys. They are live bacteria and yeasts that are beneficial to the body. Microencapsulation is a protection process where the probiotics are "coated" so that they can withstand the gastric acids and bile salts present in the body during digestion. This allows them to make it safely to the intestines where they are needed, without being destroyed. Probiotics that are NOT microencapsulated run the risk of being destroyed before they ever reach their intended destination because of the acidity of gastric juice and/or exposure to oxygen. (1)

For this reason, I choose ProBio5. Not only is it microencapsulated (with necessary enzymes to combat Candida as I mentioned before), but it also has five strains of "good guys" that make it beneficial for a variety of other reasons. Here are the strains, and the reasons I love them:

- Bacillus Coagulans: this has been known to assist with digestion, nutrient absorption, and immune function. Certain Bacillus Coagulans have even been shown to enhance T-cell response which can boost immune system health. (2)
- Lactobacillus Acidophilus: this is another strain that is beneficial for the immune system. Studies suggest it can even modulate the immune response in cancer (3) and help fight irritable bowel disease (4). It's also a "soldier" type of bacteria that fights against many different pathogens like E. Coli, Staph, Salmonella, and Candida. And it can be beneficial in

- treating/preventing/reducing vaginal infections, cold/flu symptoms, and allergy symptoms (including eczema).
- Bifidobacterium Longum: this has shown to be effective against stubborn, long-term recurrent infections like Clostridium Difficile, which I mentioned earlier (5). And research now is even suggesting it may be beneficial in preventing colon cancer. (6) Bifidobacterium can also help break down fiber, coat the inner lining of the intestines and protect it from damage, stimulate the immune system, and produce some crucial vitamins like B12, biotin, and K2.
- Lactobacillus Plantarum: this is not only valuable in fighting harmful bacteria, it can also help prevent these bad bacteria from forming colonies because it secretes substances to impede their growth. (7) It also helps repair the intestinal lining so that it can be especially useful for irritable bowel syndrome, Crohn's disease, and Colitis. (8)
- The Saccharomyces Boulardii in ProBio5 is a strain of non-pathogenic yeast. And what's interesting is that it has a unique ability to fight Candida yeast (9) as well as other widespread, harmful bacteria like H. Pylori and Clostridium Difficile (10).

Mood-Boosting Good Guys

Clearly, having a healthy gut foundation is vital for preventing infection and boosting immune function. But, as I mentioned in the last chapter, there is also a direct communication that exists between the gut and the brain. So, good gut health is also crucial for improving mood.

It all goes back to the enteric "second brain" and the Vagus Nerve. The Vagus Nerve is like a highway that stretches from the brain to the intestines, where colonies of good guys interact with the nervous system and the brain, to send and receive messages. It is also believed that inflammatory markers travel this highway, linking gut inflammation to brain inflammation. So, it's no wonder studies now show a direct correlation between gut health and mental health, and why probiotics can be a valuable tool for treating some anxiety and mood disorders (11).

The gut-brain uses more than 30 neurotransmitters, just like the brain in the head. In fact, it is estimated that 90% of mood-boosting serotonin is produced in the gut. Gut microbes also play an important role in the production of Gamma-aminobutyric acid (GABA), which is a neurotransmitter that blocks impulses between nerve cells in the brain. In other words, it provides a natural calming effect (this could explain why low levels of GABA may be linked to specific anxiety disorders).

What's more, neurons in the gut generate almost as much of the neurotransmitter dopamine as neurons in the head. Dopamine is associated with the pleasure/reward system in the brain. It helps regulate mood, behavior, sleep, cognition, motivation, decision-making, and creativity. This is why abnormalities in dopamine have long been associated with attention-deficit/hyperactivity disorder (ADHD). (12)

Because good gut microbes can produce these and other important hormones and neurotransmitters (13), probiotics can be beneficial for mood issues, too. If you could use help in this area, talk to your doctor or mental health professional about taking Plexus VitalBiome™. VitalBiome™ not only comes in a delayed-release capsule, it also contains 20 Billion Live Probiotics from eight diverse strains that are PROVEN to reduce feelings of stress and anxiety as well as reduce gastrointestinal distress. These are researched and proven strains, backed by 279 scientific studies!

In fact, the results of a preliminary in vitro human gut simulator study suggest that VitalBiome's formula may have several beneficial effects:

- Increases Lactobacillus in the Ascending Colon by 418%
- Increases Bifidobacterium in the Transverse Colon by 157%
- Increases Akkermansia in the Transverse Colon by 165%

Now, that being said, please know that Plexus VitalBiome™ is not intended to be a *replacement* for ProBio 5. On the contrary, VitalBiome is like a "sister," or companion, that can be taken _with_ ProBio 5 for added benefit. As always, discuss this possibility with your doctor before taking any new supplements.

Fermented Good Guys

In addition to taking quality probiotics like Plexus® ProBio 5 and Plexus VitalBiome™, another way to add good microbes to the microbiome is to eat fermented foods. Fermented foods go through a process of lactofermentation. During lactofermentation, natural bacteria feed on the sugar and starch in the food, which then creates lactic acid. This not only preserves the food, but it also creates enzymes, b-vitamins, Omega-3 fatty acids, and probiotics like Lactobacilli and Bifidobacteria.

Fermented foods also increase the bioavailability of vitamins and minerals; they increase the body's ability to use amino acids in protein-rich foods, and they provide antioxidants to fight free radicals.

There is one thing to keep in mind, though, when shopping for fermented foods: there is a BIG difference between fermented foods and pickled foods. In my experience as a health coach, this is a common misunderstanding. Foods that are pickled are usually just preserved in something acidic, which creates a sour flavor. They are also traditionally cooked, which destroys the beneficial bacteria and enzymes in the food. So they do NOT have the same benefits.

Fermented foods, on the other hand, are fermented using a starter, salt, and filtered water. This enables a chemical reaction to take place that creates the sour flavor. Fermentation does _not_ use pressure or heat either, but it still preserves the food and lets the bacteria on the vegetable flourish without harming them. It's important to know the difference when shopping for fermented foods so that you can read labels.

For example, let's look at pickles. Typical pickles at the grocery store are often made by just soaking cucumbers in vinegar. A "pickled" pickle will list vinegar and/or citric acid in the ingredients and probably some sort of yellow dye. They will be located on a shelf in a middle aisle of the store. Whereas a truly _fermented_ pickle will be in the refrigerator section, and the label will list only cucumbers and ingredients like salt, water, and maybe some seasonings. No vinegar, no citric acid, no dye. Also, make sure the label does not list added sugars or alcohols and look for unpasteurized, organic, and non-GMO.

Depending on the supermarket you shop at, it may be challenging to find _truly_ fermented foods. If that is the case, you may consider fermenting your own foods. This not only ensures the quality and integrity of your fermented foods, but it can prove to be much more cost-effective too. There are many great resources on the internet that go through the fermentation process step by step. One that I personally like is located at Cultures for Health. (https://www.culturesforhealth.com/learn/natural-fermentation/how-to-ferment-vegetables/)

Lastly, there is another very important thing to note regarding fermented foods: Candida suffers beware! If you have a known Candida outbreak, it is definitely essential to incorporate fermented foods into your diet, but you absolutely must start slowly to avoid possible flare-ups. I have seen many clients whose symptoms worsened because they ate too many fermented foods at the beginning of their journey.

Also, Candida sufferers should beware of kombucha. Kombucha is a popular fermented drink that contains wild strains of various yeasts. In fact, some kombucha brands have even been found to contain actual candida Albicans which could make the overgrowth worse. This should be especially concerning if you have ever experienced a sort of "buzz" after drinking kombucha.

Healthy Examples of Fermented Foods

Keto-Friendly Options:	Not-Keto-Friendly Options:
Sauerkraut	Kefir
Kimchi	Kombucha
raw cheese	Miso
apple cider vinegar	Tempeh
cured olives	Natto
certain pickles	yogurt

Feed the Good Guys!

I've already talked about how things like sugar feed harmful bacteria such as Candida yeast, and how we should stay away from these things to prevent overgrowth. Now let's talk about what feeds good bacteria. If we want an abundance of the good guys (to combat the bad guys), then we not only need to populate the gut with them, we also need to feed them and create an environment for them to flourish. The primary foods that can feed these good bacteria are prebiotics. PREbiotics feed PRObiotics.

Prebiotics are basically undigestible ingredients, mostly fibers. We don't use these fibers for energy, but the friendly bacteria in the gut DO use them. They help them grow and flourish, so they can do all the important jobs we've been talking about (like make hormones, regulate metabolism, assist the immune system, and fight pathogens). The question is, what are the best prebiotic foods to eat? Well, here are my favorites (from greatest to least):

- Raw Chicory Root: Chicory root is almost 65% fiber by weight, and much of it is inulin fiber which has been proven to stimulate the growth of Bifidobacterium (14) which is needed for digestion, preventing infection, and producing vitamins and other important chemicals.
- Raw Jerusalem Artichoke: More than ¾ of its fiber comes from inulin, and it is known to increase good bacteria in the colon specifically.
- Raw Garlic: Garlic is more than 17% fiber, 11% of which is inulin and 6% is fructooligosaccharides (FOS), and it has antioxidant effects.
- Raw Onion: Onion is more than 16% fiber, 10% of which is inulin and 6% is FOS. They have flavonoids, antioxidants, and can help boost the immune system. Red onions also have additional flavonoids called anthocyanin (pigments) which make them even more useful against free radicals.
- Raw Leeks: Leeks are part of the onion family but are a little sweeter. They are more than 11% fiber and are rich in vitamin K and vitamin C.

- Raw Asparagus: It's tough to eat raw asparagus (quite literally), but it can be fermented. It can also be chopped in a food processor or blender and sprinkled into recipes. Raw asparagus is approximately 5% fiber.
- Unripe Bananas: These have resistant starch in them, which gives them prebiotic potential. They are only about 1% fiber, but one cup of mashed unripe banana also contains more than 20% percent of your recommended daily value of potassium. Of course, these are not keto-friendly because of the sugar content.
- Apples: Apples have what is called pectin, which gives them prebiotic potential. Pectin can increase short-chain fatty acid butyrate. Butyrate has been known to feed good bacteria and decrease harmful bacteria.

As you will notice, each of these says "raw" before it. That's because cooking or even heating will destroy some of the fiber and some of the prebiotic potential. So, keep that in mind when cooking.

In addition to these foods, I would be remiss if I did not add that Plexus Slim® Microbiome Activating formula contains Xylooligosaccharides (XOS), which is a clinically-studied prebiotic fiber that has been shown to *dramatically* increase several key groups of bacteria:

- XOS increases Lactobacillus bacteria by 365 times!
- XOS increases the good Bifidobacterium bacteria by 290 times!
- XOS increases the Akkermansia microbes by 250 times! Akkermansia (aka "the metabolism bacteria") is located in the intestinal lining and helps to induce the expression of a protein called FIAF (Fasting-Induced Adipose Factor) which helps lessen fat storage! Akkermansia is also important for maintaining a healthy mucus layer in the gut lining and helps fight certain disease-causing bacteria in the intestines.

As you can see, these numbers are substantial! If I could put it this way: the Slim® XOS is for your good guys as spinach is for Popeye! Discuss this with your doctor if you are interested in trying Slim®.

The Digestive System

We've been talking about the microbiome located in the gastrointestinal (GI) tract and how important it is, but now I'd like to switch gears a little and talk about the actual GI tract itself... more specifically, the digestive process. This is another crucial aspect of gut health that makes it *foundational* to overall health.

As we know, the job of the digestive system is to take food, use it for fuel, extract nutrients out it, and deliver those nutrients to the body. Obviously, this digestive process starts in the mouth. Teeth break up food into smaller parts, then the saliva in the mouth, which contains enzymes, starts to break down that food even further. The food then goes to the throat and the esophagus where contractions push it down into the stomach.

The stomach is like a holding tank—like a mixer and grinder—with a very muscular wall. It secretes acid and very powerful enzymes to further break down the food into a paste-like substance. From there, the food goes into the small intestine. The small intestine further breaks down the paste that comes from the stomach and extracts nutrients from it.

Once the nutrients have been pulled out and absorbed through the small intestine, whatever is left over is waste, which moves on to the large intestine, also known as the colon. Through a series of contractions, this waste is pushed through the colon (sometimes over 36 hours or so) and then is eliminated from the body in a bowel movement.

Because each of these steps plays a critical role in the digestive process, I'd like to go over each of them in detail. Let's start with the mouth.

Not only do teeth break down the food but so does saliva. Saliva contains not only enzymes but also electrolytes and antibacterial compounds, etc. Approximately 30% of digestions should take place in the mouth. But what happens if it doesn't? What happens if you're a fast eater and don't chew your food well enough?

Well, you start the digestive process on the wrong foot. If that 30% of digestion doesn't take place in the mouth, then one of the later parts of the digestive process will need to make up for that (the stomach, the intestines, something). It's important not to underestimate what takes place in the mouth. The longer food is chewed, the more enzymes are released. The more enzymes that are released means, the more the food will be broken down (and the easier it will be broken down), and the more nutrients will be able to be pulled from it. In other words, the more you chew, the less is lost.

If there are larger particles that pass through that are not broken down, bacteria in the intestines will have to pick up the slack and break it down. It could start to petrify, which could lead to gas, bloating, etc.

4 Rules for Chewing

1. Take small bites! Don't overburden your digestive system by giving it large amounts of food at one time.
2. Chew food until it is almost liquified. Do not swallow large food chunks.
3. Wait to take a drink until you've swallowed your food (so that you don't inadvertently swallow chunks).

4. Stop chewing for no reason (this includes chewing gum)! Think about it. Chewing starts the release of saliva and enzymes because it anticipates the start of the digestive process. If the body begins this process, but there is no actual food to break down, then there can be too much acid present. This can potentially confuse the body so that the next time it *does* have food present, it won't know how much acid to make (because it won't know if you're chewing gum or real food).

An excellent first step in rebuilding your digestive system is to chew your food conscientiously. Start chewing longer than you usually do. Aim for a paste-like substance with no chunks!

The Stomach and GERD

After food leaves the mouth, it travels down the throat and esophagus and makes its way into the stomach. The stomach is like a holding tank—or a mixer and grinder—with a very muscular wall surrounding it. In a perfect world, the stomach secretes acid and very powerful enzymes to further break down the food into a paste-like substance so that it can be pushed down into the small intestine.

Unfortunately, for many, this process doesn't work as well as it should. Sometimes, stomach contents and stomach acid come back up into the esophagus and the throat. When stomach acid touches the lining of the esophagus, it can cause symptoms known as heartburn or acid indigestion. If this is ongoing, it can develop into what is known as Gastroesophageal Reflux Disease (or GERD).

Unfortunately, this is quite common as GERD affects between 15-30% of the U.S. population. (15) GERD then can then cause Esophagitis (inflammation in the esophagus), and also respiratory issues if stomach acid is breathed into the lungs.

Usually, treating GERD involves taking prescription acid blockers, like proton pump inhibitors. What's a proton pump? Well, remember, at the beginning of this book I talked about how the mitochondria in the cell produce energy? Well, they produce that energy (that ATP) by pumping protons across the membrane of the cell via a "proton pump."

The belief is that if you "inhibit" the pump it will reduce acid production. Less acid, they say, will alleviate symptoms. It sounds like a win-win but, in my opinion, it's not quite that simple. Proton pumps are not just in the cells in the stomach. They are in almost every cell in the body. So, if you inhibit the pump that helps the cell produce energy, you could experience decreased energy.

Maybe your GERD is so bad that you're willing to deal with increased fatigue if it means decreased reflux. But, fatigue isn't the only side effect or risk. Because proton pump inhibitors reduce stomach acid, they can change the pH of the stomach, even the PH of the intestines, which is not a good thing. This can create a breeding ground for certain types of harmful bacteria that thrive in more alkaline conditions and potentially cause an overgrowth.

Proton pump inhibitors can also reduce the absorption of some nutrients that depend on acid for absorption. This can potentially increase the risk of deficiencies (for example, vitamin B12, vitamin C, calcium, iron, and magnesium). Proton pump inhibitors inhibit the production of nitric oxide, which helps dilate blood vessels and improve blood flow (which could increase cardiovascular risk). (16) (17) They increase the risk of developing kidney disease (18), dementia (19), and Alzheimer's disease. (20)

My concern is that proton pump inhibitors still don't solve the mystery of _why_ GERD developed in the first place. Some might say GERD is a result of a defective lower esophageal valve—it doesn't close properly, and that enables acid to flow back into the esophagus. Yeah, maybe. But is that really the _origin_ of GERD? My question is: was the valve always defective or did it become defective over time and now just needs "rebuilt" somehow? These are important questions that, in my opinion, should definitely be discussed with your doctor.

If it became defective over time, then the next question is: what caused it to become defective? From what I have seen, many GERD suffers also have a bacterial overgrowth in the gut, coincidentally. Bacterial overgrowth can result in abdominal pressure, and that pressure can drive acid back upward into the esophagus. (And acid that is continuously pressured back into the esophagus, can erode the valve over time, yes.)

If you are concerned about the possible risks associated with GERD medications, or if you want to address the _origin_ of your GERD, talk to your doctor. Ask him/her about trying to rebuild your gut health with ProBio5, Slim, VitalBiome, Bio Cleanse (which I will talk more about in the next phase), and of course, a gut-friendly diet low in sugar and rich in prebiotic fibers.

The Stomach and Gastritis

One of the most common stomach issues worldwide is Gastritis (inflammation in the gastric mucosa lining of the stomach). In fact, it has been estimated that more than half of the world's population could have this disease to some extent. (21) The symptoms include pain in the upper abdominal area, sometimes accompanied by burning, belching, nausea, vomiting, and/or bloating. In some cases, the stomach lining can even become damaged which causes intense burning, stomach ulcers, and malabsorption of nutrients (essential vitamins, like vitamin B12, and micronutrients like iron, calcium, magnesium, and zinc).

The leading cause of Gastritis is a bacterial infection known as Helicobacter Pylori (aka H Pylori) which I mentioned earlier in this chapter. H Pylori often begins in childhood. The bacteria can be transmitted via saliva from infected people, or via food, water, or utensils. Because H Pylori comes from fecal matter, it is transmitted through a lack of hand-washing and unsanitary conditions, especially in underdeveloped areas. But it is not limited to those areas, because studies are now suggesting that more than 50% of the world's population is infected with H Pylori. Among those, hundreds of millions of people develop peptic ulceration during their lifetime and still tens of millions might progress to gastric cancer. (22)

Studies are showing, though, that you're not doomed if you have H Pylori. In fact, chronic gastritis can be cured with the eradication of H. pylori, and this can result in the gastric mucosa lining returning to normal. (23) But how do you treat H Pylori? Conventional treatment often involves multiple rounds of antibiotics and/or proton pump inhibitors. I've already gone over the risks associated with both, so if you share these concerns, my suggestion is to discuss them with your doctor.

You may also want to discuss natural alternatives such as ProBio5, Slim, VitalBiome, and BioCleanse because studies have shown that taking multiple strains of probiotics can eradicate H Pylori proving that good gut health is important. (24) Some people have also benefitted from drinking all-natural, home-brewed green tea, and using Lemongrass and/or Lemon Verbena essential oils. These oils have been found to be bactericidal against H. pylori in in-vitro studies. (25)

There are a few different ways to use essential oils. One, you can rub them topically on the skin (in this case, on your stomach) on top of a carrier oil such as Jojoba oil. You can also put a couple of drops of essential oils in an empty capsule and swallow it, or you can put a few drops in a glass of filtered water and drink it. However, please note that not all essential oils are created equal. You never, EVER want to ingest oils that are not certified organic and/or therapeutic grade. And it is *imperative* that you consult your doctor before ingesting any oils, especially if you have other, preexisting health conditions.

The Small Intestine

After food leaves the stomach, it travels in a paste-like form called chyme to the small intestine. The small intestine is an 18-20-foot tube coiled up in the abdominal cavity. It is divided up into three parts: Duodenum, Jejunum, and Ileum. This part of the digestive system is enormously crucial to the overall health of the body. It is foundational, and therefore, is not to be underestimated in the rebuilding attempt!

The Duodenum is the first 10-12 inches of the small intestine. It's the busiest part of the small intestine and the part where the most digestion occurs. The Duodenum receives the paste from the stomach and mixes it with enzymes from the pancreas as well as bile from the liver and gallbladder. This completely breaks down all carbs, proteins, and fats into sugars, amino acids, and fatty acids. At that point, the first phase of digestion is completed, and the mixture moves to the second part of the small intestines, called the Jejunum, through a series of contractions.

The Jejunum is where most of the absorption of nutrients occurs. Along the wall of the small intestine, there are finger-like projections, called villi, that stick out like bristles on a hairbrush. The job of the villi is to make contact, or kind of "brush" the food that passes through. Each of the villi has other bristle-like projections on it, called microvilli. It's as if each of the bristles on your hairbrush had its own bristles on the bristles. The bristles of the small intestine are called villi. The bristles on the bristles are called microvilli.

On these villi and microvilli, there are enzymes that help absorb nutrients. Sugars and amino acids are absorbed into the blood capillaries in the villi. Fatty acids are too big to fit into the blood capillaries, so they are absorbed through veins and arteries, which then transport it through the body.

After this takes place, what is left of the food moves on to the third part of the small intestine, which is Ileum. The main job of the Ileum is to absorb vitamin B12. It also reabsorbs bile salts and recycles them back to the liver. B12 is crucial for energy production, blood formation, DNA synthesis, nerve formation, etc. From there, the food moves to the colon for elimination.

Dysfunction or damage to any of these parts of the small intestine can lead to serious problems. The following are a few of the most common health issues related to the small intestine:

1. **Small Intestinal Bacterial Overgrowth (SIBO)** —SIBO is as the name implies, an overgrowth of bacteria in the small intestine. While it's normal to have some bacteria in the digestive tract, the largest amount should be in the colon, not the small intestine. When there's an overgrowth of harmful bacteria in the small intestine, it can lead to gas, bloating, pain, eczema, acne, and asthma. It can also lead to poor nutrient absorption because SIBO has been found to diminish villi and reduce the absorptive capacity of the microvilli. (26) If bacteria move up through the GI tract, it can also damage the stomach lining.
2. **Irritable Bowel Syndrome (IBS)**—IBS is an umbrella term for a broad range of digestive symptoms that cannot be otherwise diagnosed... such

as abdominal pain, constipation, diarrhea, indigestion, nausea, and gas. Interestingly, though, research now suggests that SIBO may be responsible for up to 78% of IBS cases. (27)

3. **Celiac Disease** —As I mentioned before, Celiac disease is an autoimmune disease. When sufferers eat gluten (the protein that is in wheat, rye, and barley), their body creates an immune response and then attacks the small intestine and damages the villi. This leads to poor nutrient absorption. What's interesting too is that it has been found that there is a high incidence of SIBO in celiac patients who still had symptoms after removing gluten from the diet. (28) This makes sense considering SIBO can lead to diminished villi (26), which is the main characteristic of Celiac disease.

4. **Inflammatory Bowel Disease (IBD)**—IBD is a group of two diseases, Crohn's disease, and Ulcerative Colitis, that are both characterized by chronic inflammation of the GI tract and are listed as autoimmune diseases (29). With Crohn's disease, the intestine becomes inflamed, sores develop, and often so does SIBO (30). Ulcerative Colitis is similar except that the inflammation and sores develop in the colon and rectum. IBD is believed to be caused by a combination of factors: heredity, a weakened immune system, and environmental factors such as bacteria, virus and/or toxins. But what's extremely important to note is that leaky gut syndrome is also usually present in inflammatory bowel disease. In fact, several studies show that changes in intestinal permeability can even predict IBD. (31)

Intestinal Tools

If you would like to try and rebuild your digestive system naturally, because of the above issues, make an appointment with your doctor. Ask about the Plexus tools I've mentioned in this chapter (Triplex especially) as these products contain ingredients that are often beneficial in rebalancing gut dysbiosis and addressing bacterial overgrowths (two common denominators in the above-listed issues).

However, if you have one of the diseases that are autoimmune in nature, it is very important that you go _slowly_. Ask your doctor if the Autoimmune Disease Dosing Chart (listed in the appendix), is safe for you. If your practitioner approves the dosing chart, be sure to stay in close contact with him/her so they can manage your progress and help you troubleshoot. It is not uncommon for people with autoimmune diseases to also have severe candida or dysbiosis, which can result in serious die-off symptoms. It is, therefore, _necessary_ to ease into a rebuilding strategy with ongoing help from a licensed medical professional.

Ease

It may also be worth asking your doctor about Plexus Ease because the ingredients in Ease are specifically designed to combat inflammation, which is the primary and causal issue underlying Crohn's and Colitis. <u>But please note, Plexus Ease contains green-lipped mussel and is not suitable for people with some seafood allergies.</u> Green-lipped mussel, though, has been found to have impressive anti-inflammatory properties (32) especially when it comes to IBD (33) and arthritis. (34)

Ease also contains a substantial amount of turmeric, which has been found to be anti-inflammatory in six human trials. (35) And consuming black pepper with Ease might increase the absorption of turmeric by up to 2000%. (36)

xFactor Plus

Because the small intestine is heavily involved in nutrient absorption, and intestinal issues can hinder this absorption, ask your doctor about taking Plexus xFactor Plus. We have already gone over the numerous benefits of xFactor Plus, but to recap, these are the ones most relevant to the foundation of the temple:

1. xFactor Plus contains the most bioactive and bioavailable forms of various vitamins for optimal absorption. This can be quite beneficial for those with intestinal issues and compromised absorption.
2. xFactor Plus contains methylated forms of vitamin B12 and Folate (vitamin B9) which can be beneficial for those with a dysfunctional Ileum.
3. xFactor Plus is also "microbiome activating," meaning it contains ingredients that can activate and support good gut bacteria.
4. Not only does xFactor Plus has 100% or more of the daily value (DV) of 19 essential vitamins and minerals, and more than 50 naturally occurring trace minerals, it also has a gut-protecting polyphenol blend.

The Intestinal Diet

To maintain intestinal health, it is also important to look at the ingestible things that can potentially damage the small intestine, and then stay away from those. The biggest culprits in my professional opinion are toxins (anything artificial that the small intestine is not designed to absorb), pesticides, and GMOs like soy and corn (which have a greater pesticide residue than typical plants).

The ketogenic diet can also prove beneficial for several reasons. One, ketosis naturally helps reduce inflammation, because ketone metabolism produces fewer reactive oxygen species, which are known to contribute to inflammation. (And remember, inflammation is present in most of the above listed intestinal issues.) (37)

Two, by eliminating sugar, you help starve any harmful bacteria that feed on sugar that may be present in SIBO. Some people argue that the ketogenic diet can make SIBO worse. That's because, with a "typical" keto diet, you eliminate carbs, and thereby eliminate prebiotic fibers too, which feed the good bacteria that combat the harmful bacteria.

What's more, according to Stanford microbiome researcher, Dr. Justin Sonnenburg, "when you starve these microbes, they start eating you. When you don't eat dietary fiber...you are forcing the microbes into a position where they are forced to consume the important immunological barrier in your gut." (38) But remember this *Rebuilding Your Temple* protocol does not eliminate prebiotic fibers; it increases them for the proliferation of *good* bacteria.

In fact, with the XOS prebiotics in Plexus Slim, you could be increasing them by hundreds of times. So, following this protocol you get the gut-benefits of ketosis without the risks. Also, some people with severe Chron's or Colitis have difficulty digesting an abundance of fibrous vegetables. Plexus Slim may allow them to get the necessary prebiotics without the pain associated with digestion.

Three, the keto diet eliminates wheat, which is often very important for intestinal health because wheat proteins provoke an inflammatory immune response in the GI tract. (Those who suffer from IBD and IBS may want to consider limiting dairy consumption as it too can be inflammatory and aggravate symptoms. As always, discuss this with your doctor, especially if you are low in calcium.)

References:

(1) https://www.sciencedirect.com/science/article/pii/S1978301916300171
(2) https://www.ncbi.nlm.nih.gov/pubmed/19332969
(3) https://www.ncbi.nlm.nih.gov/pubmed/22711009
(4) http://www.microbiologyresearch.org/docserver/fulltext/jmm/59/2/141.pdf?expi res=1527333279&id=id&accname=guest&checksum=DBA40980405A2F3C958502 7C11D522BF
(5) https://www.ncbi.nlm.nih.gov/pmc/articles/PMC3105609/
(6) https://www.ncbi.nlm.nih.gov/pubmed/24068536
(7) https://www.ncbi.nlm.nih.gov/pmc/articles/PMC1175894/
(8) https://www.ncbi.nlm.nih.gov/pmc/articles/PMC539443/
(9) https://www.ncbi.nlm.nih.gov/pubmed/20629753
(10) https://www.ncbi.nlm.nih.gov/pubmed/16292090/
(11) https://www.ncbi.nlm.nih.gov/pmc/articles/PMC3904694/

(12) http://journals.plos.org/plosone/article?id=10.1371/journal.pone.0183509
(13) https://www.ncbi.nlm.nih.gov/pmc/articles/PMC4259177/
(14) https://gut.bmj.com/content/66/11/1883
(15) https://www.healthline.com/health/gerd/facts-statistics-infographic#1
(16) https://www.ncbi.nlm.nih.gov/pmc/articles/PMC3838201/
(17) http://journals.plos.org/plosone/article?id=10.1371/journal.pone.0124653
(18) http://jasn.asnjournals.org/content/early/2016/04/13/ASN.2015121377
(19) https://jamanetwork.com/journals/jamaneurology/fullarticle/2487379
(20) https://www.ncbi.nlm.nih.gov/pubmed/23520537
(21) https://www.ncbi.nlm.nih.gov/pmc/articles/PMC4673514/
(22) https://www.ncbi.nlm.nih.gov/pmc/articles/PMC2841423/
(23) https://www.ncbi.nlm.nih.gov/pmc/articles/PMC4673514/
(24) https://www.ncbi.nlm.nih.gov/pubmed/22452604
(25) https://www.ncbi.nlm.nih.gov/pubmed/12752733
(26) https://www.ncbi.nlm.nih.gov/pmc/articles/PMC3099351/
(27) https://www.ncbi.nlm.nih.gov/pmc/articles/PMC3949258/
(28) https://www.ncbi.nlm.nih.gov/pubmed/12738465
(29) https://www.aarda.org/diseaselist/
(30) https://www.ncbi.nlm.nih.gov/pmc/articles/PMC2728727/
(31) https://www.ncbi.nlm.nih.gov/pmc/articles/PMC2728727/
(32) https://www.ncbi.nlm.nih.gov/pubmed/7194074
(33) https://www.ncbi.nlm.nih.gov/pubmed/15870972
(34) https://www.ncbi.nlm.nih.gov/pubmed/22366869
(35) https://www.ncbi.nlm.nih.gov/pubmed/12676044
(36) https://www.ncbi.nlm.nih.gov/pubmed/9619120
(37) https://www.ncbi.nlm.nih.gov/pmc/articles/PMC4124736/
(38) https://www.youtube.com/watch?v=TRy9A-BYmx8

Phase 5:

Rebuilding the Plumbing

Materials: Raw Veggies, Chia Seeds, Hemp Seeds, Flaxseed, Cilantro, Onions, and High-Fiber Grains

Tools: Plexus Bio Cleanse™ and Plexus Slim®

Chapter 10: Drainage and Detoxification

Let's begin Phase 5 of the temple rebuild, and work on the plumbing! In this phase, we will look at the body's detoxification system, which is very much like the drainage system of a house. It not only recycles fluids back into the body but also collects and eliminates wastes and toxins.

The drainage system in a house works behind the scenes. It isn't very noticeable— that is until it isn't working correctly—until the toilet won't flush, or the kitchen sink or bathtub won't drain. Such is the case with the temple drainage system too. You don't think much about toxin/waste elimination until constipation or toxicity occurs. Then, it quickly moves to the top of the priority list. The thing is, it should always be at the top.

The body's "plumbing" is similar to the foundation in that it is essential for overall health. If you are not eliminating waste and toxins properly, these can build up inside and lead to serious diseases, like cancer. Unfortunately, many people don't give this system the consideration it deserves. But we will, now, starting with this chapter.

The two areas I will focus on in this phase are the lymphatic system and the excretory system (skin, liver, lungs, large intestine, and kidneys). The two most apparent jobs of the excretory system are bowel movements and urination. So, we will pick up from where we left off in the last phase and talk about elimination.

After food is digested and nutrients are extracted and absorbed in the small intestine, what remains of the food is considered waste. This waste moves from the small intestine to the large intestine, also known as the colon, or the bowel. While it is called the "large" intestine, it is only about six feet long, which is much shorter than the small intestine (though it is much fatter).

Once this waste is in the colon, liquids and salts are removed from the waste and reabsorbed into the body. Vitamins (like vitamin K) are also absorbed. Then the waste makes its way to the end of the colon where it is stored until the body is ready to make a bowel movement, once or twice a day.

Constipation

Unfortunately, many people are unable to make a regular, daily bowel movement and therefore suffer from constipation. In fact, it has been estimated that more than 4 million people in the United States have frequent constipation, storing between 5 and 10 pounds of old fecal matter in their bodies. This is the most common digestive complaint in the United States, outnumbering all other chronic digestive conditions. (1)

There can be many different things that cause this—stress, nerve issues, medications, lack of fiber, thyroid problems, lack of water, too much dairy, diabetes, overuse of laxatives, inactivity, resisting the urge to go, processed food, pelvic floor disorders, GI issues, dysbiosis, or microbiome changes.

Regardless of the cause, complications associated with chronic constipation can be serious. Aside from just the discomfort associated with bloating, hemorrhoids, and fishers (tears), constipation can cause various carcinogens in the stool to become more concentrated. As these come in contact with cells that are lining the colon and rectum, it can increase the risk of developing colon cancer.

Chronic constipation can also cause toxins to be reabsorbed into the body via the colon (2) and gut microbes to become imbalanced (a reduction in good bacteria and overgrowths of harmful bacteria). (3)

Often, people turn to laxatives or extreme colon cleanses to alleviate constipation. But this comes with several risks:

1. Some herbal laxatives can cause liver damage (4) and hepatitis (5)
2. Some forms of extreme colon cleansing methods can result in cramping, abdominal pain, fullness, bloating, nausea, vomiting, perianal irritation, soreness, electrolyte imbalance, renal failure, aplastic anemia, and liver toxicity. (6)
3. Some OTC laxatives, such as MiraLax, contain Polyethylene glycol 3350 (PEG 3350), which is a petroleum-based substance made from the chemical Ethylene Glycol (EG) in antifreeze. The FDA says PEG 3350 is safe for adult consumption but also warns of possible "neuropsychiatric events." (7) It's not surprising, considering Ethylene Glycol is chemically broken down in the body into toxic compounds that affect the central nervous system, the heart, and the kidneys. (8) Additionally, PEG can destroy intestinal bacteria just as drastically as antibiotics, leading to dysbiosis which we've already discussed at length.

4. Lastly, most conventional treatments are inefficient. When rotting waste materials stay in the colon too long, they can begin to harden and stick to the colon wall. This can be a huge problem because they can form a 2-3-inch thick layer that is as hard as tire rubber, making it extremely difficult to get rid of. Laxatives and cleanses may help move waste through the colon, but rarely do they address the fecal matter on the colon wall, which can be just as problematic.

An Alternative

If you are not comfortable with conventional treatments because of the risks, ask your doctor about Plexus Bio Cleanse™. The main ingredient in Bio Cleanse is magnesium hydroxide. I've already talked extensively about the numerous benefits of magnesium on other systems, but there are even more benefits when it comes to intestinal health. Not only does it work like an antacid (magnesium hydroxide combines with hydrogen ions in stomach acids to create water and eventually neutralize stomach acid), but it also is an effective treatment for constipation. Magnesium hydroxide draws water into the colon, making the stool softer so it can be passed more easily.

What I think is also beneficial about Plexus Bio Cleanse™, though, is the *added* ingredients—namely, vitamin C, sodium bicarbonate, and the bioflavonoid complex that includes orange peel, lemon peel, and quince. Why are these important? Well, because they work synergistically with the magnesium hydroxide for increased effectiveness.

You see, this synergistic effect can break apart the magnesium-peroxide bond. This then releases ozone and peroxides into the body which can soften that thick, "tire-rubber-like plaque" on the intestinal wall that I mentioned earlier. It can also kill pathogenic microbes. The ozone and peroxides then break down even further (into oxygen), which purifies and energizes the cells in the body. The magnesium then creates a colon-flushing reaction which sends the softening plaque and dead bacteria out of the body through a bowel movement and prevents reabsorption of the toxins.

This is especially important if you are taking Plexus® ProBio 5. In my opinion, ProBio5 and Bio Cleanse should always go hand in hand, but you must talk to your doctor first. As ProBio 5 works to destroy harmful bacteria, it is important to have Bio Cleanse working simultaneously to remove those dead microbes—especially when it comes to Candida. When Candida dies, it releases all the harmful substances that were in it, which includes more than 70 toxins, like ethanol, uric acid, and acetaldehyde. It is essential to open up detoxification pathways so that the body can flush those out.

However, even though I personally consider Bio Cleanse to be one of the most valuable tools in the toolbelt, it's important to talk to your doctor before taking Bio Cleanse, especially if you are taking any medications (like statins and thyroid medications) because magnesium can interfere with their absorption.

It can also interfere with Dasatinib (Spyrcel), Delavirdine (Rescriptor), Digoxin (Digox or Lanaxin), Mycophenolate, Atazanavir, Phosphate supplements like potassium phosphate, Tetracycline antibiotics like doxycycline and minocycline, Quinolone antibiotics like ciprofloxacin or levofloxacin, Azole antifungals like ketoconazole and itraconazole.

Therefore, Bio Cleanse may need to be taken several hours apart from medications, or as your doctor sees fit.

Fiber

Another thing that helps constipation is increased fiber consumption. As I mentioned earlier, there are two kinds of fiber—soluble and insoluble. Soluble fiber helps water stay in the stool, making it softer and more comfortable to pass. Insoluble fiber adds bulk to the stool, making the colon feel full so that it begins elimination.

It's been estimated that adult women need at least 25 grams of fiber daily, and men 35 grams. This can be tricky while eating a ketogenic diet because the foods that serve as energy sources are high in fat and often low in fiber, whereas, on a non-ketogenic diet, the energy sources (carbs) already have the fiber in them (or at least they should if you are eating the right ones). It's not an impossible feat on keto, though. It just requires diligence. A few keto-friendly ways to increase fiber might be:

- Eat a big salad once every day
- Add chia seeds, hemp seeds, and/or flaxseed to your smoothies
- Add psyllium husk to your homemade, low-carb pancakes or wraps
- Have raw veggies (broccoli, celery, cauliflower) with a homemade low carb dip as your snack.

Fiber, Slim and Water

While we are on the subject of fiber, remember that Plexus Slim Hunger Control has 6,250 mg of polydextrose, a non-digestible oligosaccharide. Not only is polydextrose a low-calorie soluble fiber that takes up space in the stomach and leaves slowly (so it helps you feel full longer), it also acts as a prebiotic for good bacteria, promoting the growth of Bifidobacterium and Lactobacillus. However, Slim Hunger Control is not meant to replace the Slim Microbiome Activating formula, which has the powerful XOS prebiotics for gut health. It is offered in addition to that.

Lastly, as you can see, water is an important part of alleviating and preventing constipation, as it helps form and pass stools. So, I want to remind you again of the importance of increasing your water intake. For most people, it helps to drink half of your body weight in ounces of purified water each day.

The Lymphatic System

Another important part of the temple's "plumbing" or drainage system is the lymphatic system. The lymphatic system (which is part of the immune system) is made up of many organs, lymph vessels and lymph nodes that transport an infection-fighting fluid of white blood cells throughout the body. Its main job is to get rid of toxins, pathogens, debris from dead cells, and waste from every cell in the body. It pulls these from tissue and transports them to the blood, where the liver breaks them down before they are excreted.

There is also the glymphatic system, which is part of the lymphatic system, that mainly just works on removing toxins from the brain. The lymphatic system is highly active during sleep, but the glymphatic system does nearly ALL its work during sleep.

In fact, it's been shown that the beta-amyloid protein that is associated with Alzheimer's disease was cleared twice as fast from the brains of sleeping mice than mice that were kept awake. (9) So, needless to say, getting enough quality sleep is an important part of rebuilding your temple's plumbing and drainage system.

If this system becomes sluggish or even clogged, you can end up with toxin or waste buildup in the brain or anywhere in the body. Why is this a problem? A poorly functioning lymphatic system is a risk factor for the development of cancer, as well as other serious illnesses and chronic diseases that basically stem from a weakened immune system.

Some signs of a sluggish drainage system include headaches, swollen or aching neck, itchy or dry skin, cellulite, swollen breasts especially during menstruation, joint pain or stiffness (especially in the morning), chronic sinus issues (including sore throats and earaches), weight gain, fatigue, and brain fog.

The lymphatic system is similar to the circulatory system in that it transports important fluid through the body. The circulatory system transports blood; the lymphatic system carries lymph. However, the circulatory system has the heart which acts as a built-in pump to push the blood around. The lymphatic system does not have a pump. It relies on manual stimulation—the contraction and relaxation of the muscles and joints—to move the lymph. Therefore, a sedentary lifestyle can be very hard on the temple drainage system.

The following are ways to keep things moving through the lymphatic system:

- Ketogenic Diet: inflammation can cause lymph fluid to become trapped in the body. Therefore, because the ketogenic diet is so anti-inflammatory, it can significantly assist the lymphatic system and drainage.
- Laughter: belly laughter creates pressure in the thoracic duct (the largest lymphatic vessel in the body), which pushes lymph through lymphatic vessels, increasing both the speed and flow of lymph.
- Water: lymph is a fluid made up of water, and so the lymphatic system needs to be hydrated to function as it should. Dehydration can result in sluggish drainage or even clogged drainage.
- Sleep position: sleeping on your left side takes the pressure off the liver and can increase lymph flow, which is why many holistic practitioners call the left side of the body "the dominant lymphatic side."
- Rebounding: because jumping on a trampoline (also known as rebounding) causes the body to move against gravity, it can stimulate the lymphatic system to move lymph fluid through the vessels.
- Dry brushing: Brush the skin in long, gentle, sweeping strokes toward the heart. This helps increase lymph flow because the lymphatics are one-way valves. After brushing, take a warm shower then a cool rinse to stimulate blood circulation.
- Perspiration: sweating through the skin is one way the body eliminates toxins. For this reason, saunas can be an effective way to assist the lymphatic system.
- Exercise: not only does exercising increase sweating, but it also increases oxygen supply to tissues and cells and stimulates circulation. If the body is sedentary and does not regularly move, toxins can build up in muscles.
- Loose Clothes: tight-fitting clothes (especially around chest and arms) can restrict lymphatic vessels and hinder drainage.
- Massages and Chiropractic Care: chiropractic adjustments can increase pressure in the thoracic region which can help oxygenate cells and improve lymph flow. Foam rolling and/or massages promote the flow and drainage of lymph through the body.

Intermittent fasting

In addition to stimulating the lymphatic system (via the ways listed above), fasting or Intermittent Fasting (IF) has been known to help improve immune function, also. Fasting, as you know, simply means going a prolonged time without eating,

173

typically several hours, or a day or so. This isn't a new philosophy, as it is recorded in the Bible, and has been widely practiced by Christians for thousands of years.

You can also fast "intermittently" by following a schedule where you rotate periods of eating and fasting throughout the day. You can follow something like a 12/12, 10/14, or 8/16 schedule. In other words, if you are following the 8/16 schedule, you will eat all your macros within an 8-hour window, then you fast and eat or drink nothing (except water) for the remaining 16 hours of the day. For example, you might have breakfast at 10 AM, lunch at 1 PM, and then dinner at 5 or 6 PM. Then you fast 16 hours and do not eat anything until the next morning at 10:00 A.M., where you start all over again.

Why is this beneficial? One, initial fasting can help you get into a state of ketosis quicker (if you are attempting a ketogenic diet), and regular fasting can help you become more "fat-adapted" (meaning it can help you become a more efficient fat-burning machine).

Two, the body breaks down a substantial amount of white blood cells during periods of fasting, especially old and damaged cells. This triggers stem cell regeneration of new immune system cells. Stem cells are like chameleon cells. Given the right conditions, they not only regenerate, but they also have this fantastic ability to turn into different types of cells like muscle cells, red blood cells, brain cells, and immune cells, and take on specialized functions in the body.

Extended fasting essentially "flips a switch" for stem cells, where they go from an inactive state to the state of self-renewal, especially cells in the hematopoietic system (which includes your blood-making organs, bone marrow, and lymph nodes). They become little "builder cells" with the task of repairing and replacing worn-out or damaged tissue. During periods of fasting stem cells are quite literally "rebuilding your temple."

Research suggests that stem cells can flip this switch after 24 hours of fasting. (10) Other research shows that 72 hours of fasting (followed by a healthy, nutritionally sound diet) can actually regenerate the entire immune system! (11) In fact, this research showed prolonged fasting could even lower IGF-1 levels, which is a growth-factor hormone linked to aging, tumor progression, and cancer risk.

Additionally, fasting can help balance hunger hormones. In fact, studies show that ghrelin (which tells the body to eat) gradually DECREASED with fasting. In other words, patients were LESS hungry despite not eating. (12)

It can also help balance Leptin, the hunger hormone that tells you to stop eating. This may be especially important for those who suffer from Leptin resistance. Because Leptin is produced by fat cells, overweight people can sometimes have too much Leptin. You might think this is a good thing if Leptin says to stop eating, but actually, this overabundance can make the brain less sensitive to leptin… so it "resists," and doesn't listen to the signal to stop eating.

To increase Leptin sensitivity, therefore, it's important to lower the overabundance of Leptin. You can do this through fasting. In fact, one study showed that serum leptin levels in obese people decreased by 72% with fasting. In normal-weight people, it decreased by 64%. (13) This is also important because Leptin plays key roles in blood sugar regulation and insulin sensitivity too. (14) Though, fasting by its very nature causes the body to secrete less insulin because there is not a steady supply of sugar, which can also increase insulin sensitivity in those with insulin resistance, regardless of Leptin levels.

Additionally, fasting can help improve cardiovascular health, lower blood pressure, improve cholesterol; decrease inflammation, improve stress response, and reduce free radical damage. (15)

The longer the fast, the more benefits it can potentially have (up to a few days for most people). However, it's important to be smart about fasting. If you are accustomed to eating often, do not just start a prolonged fast out of the blue. Talk to your doctor. You may want to ease into it. Perhaps you may want to start with a 12/12 schedule and work your way up to an 8/16 schedule. Then maybe you will ready to try a full 24 hour fast. Again, please do not jump into an extreme fast without first consulting your doctor, especially if you have known health issues such as those below. While fasting can be beneficial for many, it is certainly NOT for everyone.

- Adrenal Fatigue— going 16-18 hours without eating can tax your adrenal glands. The adrenals help maintain blood sugar levels between meals, and so weak adrenals may not be able to support fasting, which could result in blood sugar issues.
- Stress—along those same lines, it's important to note that cortisol can go up during fasting. Fasting is a stress to the body, and if too much stress (and too much cortisol) is already a problem for you, then fasting may not be right for you at this point.
- Hypoglycemia and/or Prediabetes—fasting lowers sugar quickly, and if there is already too much insulin present, that can lower sugar even more, which can create hypoglycemia.

So, even though I personally am a huge fan of fasting, I do not suggest trying to fast for an extended time unless you first seek the advice of a medical doctor who approves it is right for you.

Heavy Metals

Unfortunately, detoxification can sometimes be difficult, especially if you are trying to get rid of heavy metals. While many rarely consider heavy metals, most of us are exposed to these every day, in a variety of ways:

Water

There is a layer of sediment in the Earth that contains arsenic, which is highly toxic to humans. This arsenic can potentially make its way from the ground into drinking water. It can also come from crops using pesticides with arsenic, or areas near coal-fired power plants, where arsenic and mercury are byproducts. This is especially problematic for people who get their water from private wells and do not have their water tested, but it can also affect those who do not have wells.

The allowable arsenic level has been a matter of debate in the U.S. While the EPA has lowered the limit in recent years, there have been complaints that an even lower limit is needed, but that it would be too expensive for water companies to comply with. (16) Other metals such as lead, copper, cadmium, and mercury have also been found in various drinking water sources.

Food

Many types of fish (especially shark, mackerel, and swordfish) have been found to contain mercury and other heavy metals. However, research has shown that the fish muscles (which humans typically eat) have the lowest concentrations of the metals, and the gills have the highest levels. (17) Rice can also absorb arsenic from irrigation water, soil, and cooking water, as can some grains and vegetables (18).

What's more, according to two studies, almost half of all tested commercial high-fructose corn syrup contained mercury. (19) Mercury cell chloralkali chemicals are often used to make dyes like FD&C Yellow 5 and FD&C Yellow 6 too. Also, chickens are often fed an arsenic-based chicken feed. The purpose is to make them grow faster, kill parasites, and make the color of meat look more appetizing. This is just one more reason why it is best to eat only organic, cage-free, free-range chicken.

Dental Fillings

Standard amalgam dental fillings (also known as silver fillings) are a mixture of heavy metals. Approximately 50% is elemental mercury, bound together with silver, copper, and tin. (20) This equates to approximately 1,000 mg of mercury in one amalgam filling, which has been estimated to be nearly one million times more mercury than what is in contaminated seafood! (21) Some argue that the fillings are bound together so they cannot leak and are therefore harmless.

However, others argue that every time you chew, mercury vapor is released (which can actually be tested for and measured at the tip of the tooth's root). According to licensed osteopathic physician and New York Times bestselling author, Dr. Mercola, "Once released from an amalgam-filled tooth, mercury in the form of nonreactive mercury vapor goes from your mouth to your lungs, then to your brain via your bloodstream. A common enzyme in your body called catalase converts (oxidizes) mercury vapor into the 'Hg2plus' form, which is VERY toxic, and traps it inside your cells. Once here, it is very difficult for your body to remove it." (21)

Still not convinced? Well, research has shown that those with multiple fillings had about 150% more mercury in their blood than those without fillings. (22) Also, amalgam fillings contain silver and tin, too, so there are multiple metals that the body is exposed to. If you are concerned about your amalgam fillings, talk to your doctor and/or your dentist.

Cigarettes

A study conducted by Johns Hopkins Bloomberg School of Public Health found that toxic heavy metals are leaking from many e-cigarettes into vapors. (23) Metals like cadmium, lead, and nickel were present in all brands tested. The primary source of the metals, the researchers believe, is the coil that heats the liquid and creates the aerosol, which is commonly called the "vapor."

This is concerning, especially for young people, because it has been estimated that the use of e-cigarettes among high school students has increased 900 percent in recent years. (23) Heavy metal exposure is not limited to e-cigarettes, though, as many tobacco cigarettes also contain the same heavy metals, as well as arsenic. (24) Even smokeless tobacco has been found to contain toxic metals.

Occupations

If you work in certain types of professions, you're at higher risk too – that includes welders, lab workers, painters, dental occupations, metalworkers, engravers, photographers, potters, printers, cosmetic workers and more.

Household Products

One of the most common and overlooked sources of heavy metal exposure in the home is cookware. For example, stainless steel pots and pans can leach nickel and chromium into foods during cooking. (25) Enameled cookware can also be concerning because some of the ceramic enamels used can contain non-stick chemicals and heavy metals. Aluminum also leaches into food from aluminum cookware. Even though the amount is believed to be less than some other products, I still advise using caution because aluminum is a known toxin to the body.

What's more, it can have an accumulative effect because we are exposed to aluminum through many other things such as some antacids, buffered aspirin, cans, juice pouches, baking powder, self-rising flour, salt, baby formula, coffee creamers, processed foods, toothpaste, and nasal spray. And while it is not a metal, the chemical Perfluorooctanoic acid (PFOA) present in Teflon cookware has been found in animal studies to cause several types of tumors and neonatal death and may have toxic effects on the immune, liver, and endocrine systems. (26)

Other household products that often contain metals are: chemical cleaners, aluminum foil, some plastic toys, batteries, old lead paint, and synthetic rubber.

Beauty Products

It's something most women do not think about—how toxic their beauty products could be. However, if you are serious about rebuilding your temple, it absolutely must be looked at. Not only are there numerous harmful chemicals in various cosmetics, but there are often heavy metals too. The FDA mandates that products must stay within limits—Arsenic: Not more than 3 ppm, Lead: Not more than 20 ppm, Mercury: Not more than 1 ppm (27).

But again, what I find concerning is the accumulative effect. Most women do not use just one beauty product (one makeup product, one lotion, one facial serum, one deodorant or one antiperspirant, etc.). They use multiple. Every. Single. Day. So even though each product stays within the FDAs limits, it is the number of products used by consumers (and the *cumulative* exposure) that is most alarming to me.

Vaccines

Aluminum is added to many different vaccines as an adjuvant, so vaccines will produce a stronger antibody response and be more protective. These vaccines include DTaP, DTaP-IPV, DTaP-HepB-IPV, DTaP-IPV/Hib, Hep A, Hep B, HPV, PCV13, Td, and Tdap. (28) Thimerosal is a mercury-based preservative used in vaccines to prevent contamination in a multi-dose vial when individual doses are drawn from it. (14) It's found in vaccines such as Td and the flu vaccine. (28)

According to Dr. Mark Hyman, M.D., "thimerosal is quickly converted to ethyl mercury in the body, where it moves rapidly from your blood to your brain." (29) And this is not a small exposure. It has been found that, in the first six months of life, a child can be exposed to 187.5 micrograms of mercury via vaccines, even though according to the EPA, the "safe" daily level of mercury exposure for a two-month-old infant is about 0.5 micrograms. (29)

If you are concerned about heavy metal exposure, or if you know that you already have high levels of heavy metals present in you, you should discuss these concerns with your doctor before receiving vaccinations.

What makes heavy metal exposure so concerning to me is the damaging effects they can have on human health. For example, mercury is a well-known neurotoxin believed to cause various neurological or psychiatric disorders such as autism spectrum disorders, Alzheimer's disease, Parkinson's disease, epilepsy, depression, mood disorders, and tremors. (30) In fact, in 1997, research found that mercury vapor inhalation by animals produced a molecular lesion in the brain similar to lesions seen in 80% of Alzheimer diseased brains. (31)

Also, animal studies have linked aluminum exposure to mental issues (behavioral, neuropathological, and neurochemical) and have also shown that aluminum negatively affects mitochondrial function (32) and attacks the central nervous system. (33) What's more, a brain autopsy study of elderly people found them to have aluminum levels 20 times higher than a middle-aged group. (34)

It's important to understand that metals such as arsenic, cadmium, lead, and mercury are toxic metals. They have absolutely no positive role in human health and are known to contribute to chronic disease. In fact, they can cause severe toxicity in many organ systems because they bind in tissue, create oxidative stress, affect endocrine function, block water flow through cells, and interfere with functions of essential minerals like magnesium and zinc. (35)

Other metals like aluminum, silver, and tin are technically not toxic metals, as long as they remain at very small amounts. But, if these metals accumulate in higher concentrations because of regular on-going exposure, then poisoning and serious damage can occur.

It often doesn't take very much exposure, either. In fact, it's being discovered that some metals are causing damage at what was once considered a safe level. For example, childhood lead exposure is now found to cause a decrease in IQ at a blood level below 2 µg/dL. The blood lead level at which the US Centers for Disease Control recommends investigation is 5 µg/dL. And metal detox therapies aren't recommended until the blood level reaches 45 µg/dL or above. (35)

Additionally, some of these metals are bio-accumulative, meaning they accumulate in the body over time. They are called "heavy" because they remain in the body for an extended time, often years. This happens because the body stores them in fat tissue as a way to keep them away from organs and prevent damage.

This is why heavy metals are also called "fat-soluble toxins." This makes them very difficult to get rid of even with a very well-functioning immune system.

It's important, therefore, to be aware of the symptoms of possible heavy metal toxicity. You may have metal buildup if you have "rebuilt" nearly every other temple system and still suffer from things such as:

- Confusion
- Abdominal pain
- Memory Problems
- Heart problems
- Brain Fog
- Numbness
- Nausea
- Central nervous system dysfunction
- Light-headedness
- Headaches
- Weakness and fatigue
- Achy joints and muscles
- Diarrhea
- Anemia
- Thyroid issues

If this is concerning to you, ask your doctor about having blood, urine, or hair testing done to determine if metals are the cause of your symptoms. If they are, then what? What can you do if you suffer from heavy metal toxicity? First, see your doctor again. Below are some possible detoxing tools that you may want to discuss with him or her.

Tools That Assist Detoxification

Plexus xFactor Plus

There are a few ingredients found in xFactor Plus that have been found to be beneficial in heavy metal detoxification. The first one is Chlorophyll. Chlorophyll is the green pigment in plants. What makes it most remarkable here is that chlorophyll is considered an important "chelate" for the body. Chelation is a process where heavy metal atoms bind to organic compounds (like those in chlorophyll) and are removed from the body, like a taxi service for toxins. Chlorophyll even can bind to and remove some of the most toxic heavy metals such as mercury. For this reason, xFactor Plus could be a very valuable tool for those with amalgam (aka "silver") fillings.

xFactor Plus also contains 150% of the recommended daily value of selenium. Selenium is sort of a mercury magnet. It binds to it and then neutralizes it so that it is not absorbed by the body and gets flushed out of the system. (36) (37) Selenium even binds mercury on a one-to-one basis (one selenium molecule can bind one mercury molecule).

Plexus Slim

Plexus Slim contains an ingredient called Alpha Lipoic Acid (ALA). ALA is not only water-soluble but also fat-soluble so it, too, can be beneficial in the detoxification of metals. In fact, it's been found that ALA can enter the cell membrane and reach high concentrations in 30 seconds. Once there, it can "trap" heavy metals and prevent cellular damage. And because ALA reaches all areas of the CNS and peripheral nervous system, and crosses the blood-brain barrier, it could be especially helpful because the fatty tissue of the brain readily accumulates lead and mercury. (38)

Plexus Bio Cleanse

Magnesium is the primary ingredient in Plexus Bio Cleanse. Magnesium supports detoxification systems because it helps produce ATP energy, which is needed for cells to pump out toxins before, during, and after they accumulate. This includes heavy metal toxins such as aluminum, mercury, lead, cadmium, beryllium, and nickel. (39) And according to Dr. Carolyn Dean, author of *"The Magnesium Miracle,"* magnesium appears to competitively inhibit the uptake of lead and cadmium, especially when they are found together. (40)

Plexus Body Cream

Plexus Body Cream contains two ingredients that I believe are also very important when it comes to heavy metal detox. The first is spirulina algae. Several studies show that spirulina is an effective chelating ingredient to remove arsenic, mercury, lead, and other heavy metals as well as radioactive substances. (41) Perhaps this is because spirulina has very high concentrations of chlorophyll which I already mentioned is a natural chelate.

The other beneficial ingredient in Plexus Body Cream is activated charcoal. Activated charcoal has a porous surface and a negative electric charge, so positive-charged toxins (such as mercury, lead, and cadmium) can bind with it.

Using Plexus Body Cream topically on the skin, followed by time spent in a sauna, could help to draw toxins out of pores even quicker. As always, talk to your doctor before implementing any new detoxification strategies or taking new supplements.

Certain foods have also been found to assist in the detoxification of heavy metals. Perhaps the most effective is an algae known as Chlorella, which is often sold as a supplement. What makes chlorella so beneficial is that it contains high concentrations of chlorophyll, which gives it its vibrant green color. It also contains B vitamins, magnesium, zinc, iron, and protein. When looking for a chlorella supplement, make sure to buy "cracked cell wall chlorella" or "broken wall chlorella." Chlorella has a tough cellular wall which makes it hard to digest. A broken or cracked version makes it more absorbable in the body.

Cilantro is also beneficial because it not only binds to heavy metals, it also mobilizes them for easier excretion. It also helps assist the liver in detoxification and can be used as an expectorant.

Onions, garlic, and shallots are known as allyl sulfides. They increase glutathione (one of the body's most important antioxidants), and the promote genes containing antioxidant response elements.

N-Acetyl-Cysteine (NAC) is produced in from the amino acid cysteine. As a sulfur-containing amino acid, it possesses two potential binding sites for metals.

In addition to these "at home" detox/chelation strategies, you can also discuss a more intense chelation therapy with your doctor. Chelation is offered as an alternative medicine practice where a chemical solution called EDTA (ethylenediaminetetraacetic acid) is injected into the bloodstream to bind with the metals. The EDTA then transport the metals to the kidneys, and they are eliminated through urine. This can be a very effective form of treatment, but it can have risk factors and side effects given the burden that is put on the kidneys. So, it is important to find an experienced practitioner who can help you through these if they arise.

Address the Root Cause

While these strategies can be very helpful in ridding the body of heavy metals, what is most important is addressing the root cause of the exposure. If your roof is leaking, you don't just focus on wiping up water on the floor. You have to stop the leak, then wipe up the water. The same is true here. It's important to determine where your exposure is coming from first. How are toxins or heavy metals making their way into your body? Is it through dental fillings, beauty products, unfiltered drinking water? You must stop (or at least drastically limit) that exposure for detoxification to be completely effective.

If you are considering having your amalgam fillings removed, you must work with an experienced and qualified (sometimes holistic) dentist who understands the risk factors and who will work cautiously and carefully to mitigate re-exposure. A careful removal procedure often involves a pre-consultation, preliminary lab work, proper ventilation, oxygen masks, a dental dam, and a high-powered vacuum. Post-procedure chelation therapy is typically part of the process also. However, this is something you may need to talk to your doctor about, not your dentist. In my experience, most dentists do not typically get involved in chelation therapies.

Regardless, it is important to discuss the procedure at length with your dentist beforehand so there are no surprises that day. If none of these precautions will be taken, you could request that they are done or look for a different dentist. Have patience, though, as sometimes this is a lengthy process... but worth the time.

*** *Important Note: when attempting any of these strategies for heavy metal detoxification, it is important to start slow, and* work closely with an experienced doctor. *I cannot stress this enough! Many of these tools can help "mobilize" metals for removal, which draws them out of their hiding places in fat storage. If they are not excreted quickly or thoroughly enough, they could re-toxify the body during the detoxification attempt. Do NOT try detoxification of heavy metals without professional medical assistance.*

References:

(1) https://www.ncbi.nlm.nih.gov/pubmed/2910654
(2) https://www.ncbi.nlm.nih.gov/pmc/articles/PMC2224051/?page=1
(3) https://www.ncbi.nlm.nih.gov/pubmed/25073603
(4) https://www.ncbi.nlm.nih.gov/pubmed/15956233
(5) https://www.ncbi.nlm.nih.gov/pubmed/19925744
(6) http://e-lactancia.org/media/papers/ColonLimpieza-FamPrac2011.pdf
(7) https://www.fda.gov/Drugs/GuidanceComplianceRegulatoryInformation/Surveillance/AdverseDrugEffects/ucm295585.htm
(8) https://www.cdc.gov/niosh/ershdb/EmergencyResponseCard_29750031.html
(9) http://science.sciencemag.org/content/342/6156/373
(10) https://www.cell.com/cell-stem-cell/fulltext/S1934-5909(18)30163-2
(11) https://www.cell.com/cell-stem-cell/fulltext/S1934-5909(14)00151-9
(12) https://idmprogram.com/fasting-ghrelin-fasting-29/
(13) https://www.ncbi.nlm.nih.gov/pubmed/8784108
(14) https://www.ncbi.nlm.nih.gov/pmc/articles/PMC3602983/
(15) https://www.sciencedirect.com/science/article/pii/S0104423013000213
(16) https://www.sciencedirect.com/science/article/pii/S0048969716313407
(17) https://www.sciencedirect.com/science/article/pii/S2314808X14000256
(18) https://onlinelibrary.wiley.com/doi/pdf/10.1111/1541-4337.12068
(19) http://www.washingtonpost.com/wp-dyn/content/article/2009/01/26/AR2009012601831.html?noredirect=on
(20) https://www.fda.gov/medicaldevices/productsandmedicalprocedures/dentalproducts/dentalamalgam/ucm171094.htm

(21) https://articles.mercola.com/sites/articles/archive/2012/04/07/dangers-of-mercury-contamination.aspx
(22) https://www.ncbi.nlm.nih.gov/pmc/articles/PMC4144270/
(23) https://www.sciencedirect.com/science/article/pii/S0013935116306995?via%3Dihub
(24) https://www.ncbi.nlm.nih.gov/pmc/articles/PMC3924441/
(25) https://www.ncbi.nlm.nih.gov/pmc/articles/PMC4284091/
(26) https://www.ncbi.nlm.nih.gov/pmc/articles/PMC2920088/
(27) https://www.fda.gov/Cosmetics/ProductsIngredients/PotentialContaminants/ucm452836.htm#learned
(28)
https://www.cdc.gov/vaccines/pubs/pinkbook/downloads/appendices/B/excipient-table-2.pdf
(29) https://www.cdc.gov/vaccines/hcp/patient-ed/conversations/downloads/vacsafe-thimerosal-color-office.pdf
(30) http://drhyman.com/blog/2010/05/19/how-to-rid-your-body-of-mercury-and-other-heavy-metals-a-3-step-plan-to-recover-your-health/
(31) https://www.ncbi.nlm.nih.gov/pmc/articles/PMC3462706/
(32) http://library.iaomt.org/document/how-mercury-causes-brain-neuron-degeneration
(33) https://www.ncbi.nlm.nih.gov/pubmed/19568732
(34) https://www.ncbi.nlm.nih.gov/pubmed/19436852
(35) https://www.ncbi.nlm.nih.gov/pubmed/12214020
(36) https://www.ncbi.nlm.nih.gov/pmc/articles/PMC3654245/
(37) https://www.ncbi.nlm.nih.gov/pubmed/698281
(38) https://www.ncbi.nlm.nih.gov/pubmed/363410
(39) http://www.altmedrev.com/archive/publications/7/6/456.pdf
(40) Sircus, Mark, Ac., OMD. *Transdermal Magnesium Therapy* (2007), page 97
(41) Dean, Carolyn, MD, ND. *The Magnesium Miracle* (2007 ed.), page 186
(42) https://www.ncbi.nlm.nih.gov/pubmed/?term=spirulina+heavy+metal

Phase 6:

Rebuilding Air Quality

Materials: Raw Fruits and Vegetables, Filtered Water

Tools: Plexus Bio Cleanse™

Chapter 11: Eating for a Balanced pH

Congratulations! You are moving on to another phase in the temple rebuild! Even though Phase 6 might be the shortest phase of this book, please don't think it is less important than other phases—because it is not.

Let's look at the house example again. Another important part of any home renovation is to address air quality. There are countless things that can diminish or taint the oxygen in a home. Maybe your furnace or vacuum filter is dirty, or you have mold particles, dust or other allergens circulating in the air. These could cause serious health problems, as you know.

Well, this is true for the temple also. There are numerous things that can affect the oxygenation of the body. We call this oxygenation the body's pH. pH is short for "potential of hydrogen." It measures how acidic or alkaline the body's fluids and tissues are. It is measured on a scale from 0 to 14, with the lower number being more acidic, and the higher number more alkaline. A pH of 7 is perfectly neutral.

Now, what does this have to do with the body and overall health?

Well, the human body is approximately 65-70% water (H_2O) which, as we know, is made up of hydrogen and oxygen. This water is mostly located within the cells, but it is also located outside cells in things like lymph fluid and blood. When there is an equal amount of oxygen and hydrogen, then the pH of this fluid is neutral (or 7.0). When there is more oxygen than hydrogen, it's alkaline (7.1 and above). When there's more hydrogen than oxygen, it's acidic (6.9 and below).

To put it into perspective, a neutral reading of 7.0 means there is ten times more oxygen available to cells than an acidic reading of 6.0. So, clearly, a healthy pH level for the body is slightly alkaline—a pH of about 7.36.

Why is this important? Why are we going to focus on this in Phase 6? Because an overly acidic body is an unhealthy body. When the body is overly acidic, it creates an environment where illness, bacteria, and yeast thrive! It's essentially a breeding ground for disease! Every single person who gets cancer has an acidic body. But, on the flip side, disease CANNOT take root or survive in a well-oxygenated environment with a balanced pH.

So, the goal of this phase is to give our cells more oxygen! We do this by ridding our diets of acidic foods and introducing more alkalizing foods and supplements. There are also lifestyle factors that influence the body's pH that we will discuss as well.

Balance, Balance, Balance

Below are two food charts showing the pH value of various foods. As I said, we want to start decreasing the acid-forming foods and increasing the more alkaline ones. See below.

ALKALINE-FORMING FOODS

MOST ALKALINE-FORMING	MORE ALKALINE-FORMING	SLIGHTLY ALKALINE-FORMING	NEUTRAL (Approx 7.0)
Raw Spinach	Garlic	Lima Beans	Raw Seeds:
Wheat Grass	Green Beans	Navy Beans	-Pumpkin
Raw Kale	Chives	Brussel	Seeds
Raw Broccoli	Almonds	Sprouts	-Sesame
Raw Celery	Avocados	Fresh Soy	Seeds
Raw Asparagus	Green Tea	Beans	-Fennel
Raw Cucumber	Raw Peas	Goat Milk	Seeds
Raw Cauliflower	Squash	Goat Cheese	-Sunflower
Red Cabbage	Sweet Potato	Whey	Seed
Raw Onions	Most Lettuce	Chestnuts	Olive Oil
Stevia	Beets	Mushrooms	Primrose Oil
Lemons	Red Raddish	Cooked	Butter
Limes	Flaxseed Oil	Veggies	Raw Milk
Grapefruit	Dates	Fresh Corn	Raw Goat
Watermelon	Pears	Bell Peppers	Milk
Papaya	Apples	Olives	Most Tap
Alfalfa	Tomatoes	Bananas	Water
Herbal Teas	Lemongrass	Pineapples	Barley
	Parsley	Wild Rice	Coconut Oil
	Melons	Millet	Fish Oil
	Dates	Amaranth	
	Figs	Quinoa	

187

Vegetable Juices Seaweeds Rhubarb Collard Greens Lemon Water Dandelion	Maple Syrup Cayenne Pepper Raw Eggplant Grapes	Chicory Cherries Coconut Water Honey Green Cabbage	Sprouted Ancient Grains Barley

ACID FORMING FOODS

NEUTRAL (Approx 7.0)	SLIGHTLY ACID-FORMING	MORE ACID-FORMING	MOST ACID-FORMING
Raw Seeds: -Pumpkin Seeds -Sesame Seeds -Fennel Seeds -Sunflower Seed Olive Oil Primrose Oil Butter Raw Milk Raw Goat Milk Most Tap Water Barley Coconut Oil Fish Oil Sprouted Ancient Grains Barley	Molasses Walnuts Blueberries Cranberries Raspberries Strawberries Plums Oranges Sprouted Wheat Brown Rice Venison Cold Water Fish Spelt Lentils Agave Raw Macadamia Raw Brazil Nuts Processed Honey Cashews Ketchup	Organ Meats Liver Soy Milk Rice Cakes Rye Bread Regular Milk Oysters Turbinado Sugar Coffee Buckwheat Oats Pecans Skinless Potatoes White Sugar Brown Sugar Deli Meat Peanuts Canned Fruit Poultry Popcorn Chocolate Tomato Sauce Canned Fruit	Cheese NonOrganic Wheat White Flour Ice Cream Beer/Wine Hard Liquor Soft Drinks Fruit Juice Vinegar Pickled Pickles Pork/Beef/Lamb Tobacco e-Cigarettes Artificial Sweeteners Carbonated Drinks Microwaved Food Processed Food Canned Food Soy Sauce Sweetened Coffee Drinks Pepperoni

	Soft-Cooked Eggs Yogurt Cottage Cheese	Mustard Bottled Water	Bacon Sausage Salami

Some of this might seem confusing at first because foods you might think are acidic are not listed in an acidic column. Here's the thing: you have to think of whether the food is acid–FORMING or alkaline–FORMING, not where the food itself falls on the pH scale.

What I mean is, even though we think of citrus foods as acidic, fruits like lemons are actually alkalizing because when they are consumed, they break down and donate alkaline mineral salt compounds like citrates and ascorbates. In other words, they taste acidic, but they contribute to an alkaline environment in your body. And that's primarily what we're going for.

Similarly, some foods that we might typically think of as mild are actually acid-forming when we consume them. Grains and milk are two examples. So, it's not so much the pH of the food as it goes into our bodies, that is important here. It's the RESULTANT pH once the food is broken down. This is dictated by the residues left behind after the nutrients are broken-down, particularly sulfates and phosphates. So, it takes a little getting used to, in terms of "seeing" your food as the _resulting_ pH, not the actual pH... but you'll get the hang of it.

And the rule of thumb: all processed food is acid causing. Processed food creates an acidic body, regardless of the kind. So, take that into consideration, too. Again, the above charts are just to help you BALANCE your diet. It's not that you can never eat anything from the Acid-Forming chart. It's that you should be eating far more from the alkaline list.

In my opinion, a diet solely from the acidic chart is a body asking for disease. Evaluate where most of your daily calories fall currently and then aim for an 80/20 rule. Try to eat at least 80% of your diet from the alkaline list, and no more than 20% from the acidic list.

Now, perhaps you are trying the keto diet, and you're looking at the above chart thinking, _"Oh no! I already gave up carbs, but now I have to give up these too!?"_ Please understand the keyword in this phase is "balance." By including this chart, I am not saying you can never eat dairy again because it's in an acidic column. No, I'm saying, look for natural, raw, unprocessed or unpasteurized dairy. Then, balance it with alkalizing foods. For example, if you do eat cheese, eat it with some raw organic spinach and fresh tomatoes. Or if you do eat beef, eat it with a large garden salad packed full of raw veggies.

Also, consider your overall daily ratio. Try to eat more alkaline foods and less acidic ones throughout the day. The primary goal is to start taking steps away from acidity. And you can ease into this, friends. Maybe start by decreasing meat consumption. Instead of having beef and chicken 6-7 days a week, try eating more salmon, tuna, cod, and halibut. Or at the very least, begin to eat organic meat which we talked about in Phase 4. These options are far less acidic than traditional beef and chicken.

This phase is especially important for those on a ketogenic diet. If you've gone keto, it can be easy to unintentionally consume a lot of acidic foods like bacon, sausage, and cheese, if you are not paying attention. I think this is why keto gets so many haters from time to time. The keto diet is NOT to be confused with a bacon and cheese diet.

Testing Your pH

If you are wondering where you are at in terms of acidity, you can check your pH using over the counter urine strips. Your pH fluctuates throughout the day, though so it may be best to test a couple of times a day to get a "big picture" view. You ideally want to be slightly alkaline, between 7.36 to 7.45, for optimal health. The best time to test your pH is about an hour before a meal or two hours after a meal. Discuss your body's pH and testing with a doctor. You can get test strips at your local drug store or on Amazon.com.

Non-Food Factors

Now, let's talk about other factors that influence the body's pH, aside from just the foods we eat.

Stress

Yep, you read that correctly. Stress affects your pH. Here's how it works. The adrenal glands produce hundreds of different hormones. One of those is the stress hormone, cortisol. What does this have to do with pH? After stress hormones are released and used for the "fight or flight" response, they can actually ferment and create an acid pH in the body. This is why some people, who are prone to headaches, often have a stressful situation just before the headache. The adrenals dump out hormones that cause acidosis, which can cut down the oxygen supply to the brain and nervous system, eating up hydrogen. Then comes another headache due to a drop in pH.

Sleep

One of the most therapeutic actions the body takes while we sleep is to bind and eliminate acid. Alkaline minerals such as calcium, sodium, potassium, and magnesium bind to acids (thus neutralizing them) allowing these to be excreted by the kidneys. The less you sleep, the less acid you eliminate. In some people, lack of sleep can also cause the stomach to produce an excess of hydrochloric acid. This excess acid must be neutralized, which creates an even higher demand for your body's precious mineral reserves. So, this is another friendly reminder to GET YOUR ZZZZZs.

Smoking

As you know, smoking has many unhealthy consequences for the body. Concerning acid and alkaline balance, the strong chemicals and toxins in cigarettes have a very acidic effect on the body. The lungs, along with the kidneys, are the main toxin-eliminating organs. Smoking not only loads the body with acid-forming toxins, but it also weakens the lungs, hampering the body's ability to eliminate toxins through expiration (breathing out). It's impossible to balance the body's pH while smoking, which means you dramatically increase your risk of cancer and other diseases. (This also goes for chewing tobacco which very acid-forming, too.)

Exercise

Moderate exercise is alkalizing to the body because it increases the oxygen flow in the blood, tissues, and organs. It also stimulates the burning and elimination of acid wastes from the body. So, a lack of exercise can contribute to the accumulation of acids in the body. BUT it's also important to note that exercising past the point of exhaustion can create acidity because of lactic acid build-up.

Water

Drinking enough water is also an important factor in balancing your pH. Water is necessary to wash acid wastes from the body's tissues, and not drinking enough water can be another cause of acidity. It's not enough to just drink half your body weight in ounces each day. The type of water you drink can also affect the pH balance in the body.

Ideally, water should be filtered to remove chlorine, ammonia, heavy metals, inorganic chemicals, pesticides, bacteria and remnants of eroding piping. Reverse osmosis is also effective at filtering tap water in the home. However, some of the filters used in reverse osmosis are so fine that they also filter out all of the beneficial alkaline minerals leaving the water slightly acidic (pH of 6.5 rather than a neutral 7.0). If this is the case for you, you may want to add a re-alkalizing/mineralizing filter to your reverse osmosis system.

Some popular name brand filters can also be used to filter out chlorine and some contaminants. Often, they are not as thorough as reverse osmosis, though, and do not filter fluoride. These usually do not filter naturally occurring minerals, though, so there isn't a need to re-mineralize water after filtration.

Also, be careful with bottled water as it too is slightly acid-forming. If you're not convinced, watch this video: https://youtu.be/LO0h_1-eT10

Beauty Products

Toxins and chemicals found in beauty products dramatically affect the body's pH! It has been estimated that the average woman puts about 515 synthetic chemicals on her body every single day without even knowing it. From lotions, hair care, makeup, fragrance, you name it. (1) This is alarming because more than 60% of what we put onto our skin is absorbed into the body. It goes directly into the bloodstream in most cases. Why is this bad? Because many of these chemicals are toxic. The European Union has banned over 1,300 chemicals found in cosmetics. But the FDA has only banned eight and has restricted three.

Oxygenation Tools

In addition to staying away from acidic foods and making alkalizing lifestyle choices, there are tools that you can use to potentially help increase oxygenation in the body—like Plexus Bio Cleanse™.

As I've already mentioned, Bio Cleanse™ contains magnesium which is an alkalizing mineral. It also is an electrolyte that helps keep the body hydrated. And remember, hydration is an important factor in balancing your pH. What's more, Bio Cleanse™ contains magnesium hydroxide which can neutralize excess acid, (1) alkalizing sodium bicarbonate (baking soda), and a bioflavonoid complex of orange (peel), lemon (peel), and quince (whole fruit).

Not only do bioflavonoids have antioxidant power, as I mentioned before, these particular bioflavonoids come from citrus fruits like lemons which are alkalizing in the body. Bio Cleanse™ also contains vitamin C, which is also called ascorbic acid. You'd think that because it's called an acid that it would make your body more acidic, but it actually does the opposite. Once inside the body, you burn the acids from ascorbic acid and are left with an alkaline end-product.

Also, bioflavonoids have been used in alternative medicine to enhance the action of vitamin C, so again, the Bio Cleanse ingredients work synergistically together. As always, talk to your doctor before taking any new supplements.

References:

(1) https://www.huffingtonpost.com/entry/synthetic-chemicals-skincare_us_56d8ad09e4b0000de403d995

(2) https://pubchem.ncbi.nlm.nih.gov/compound/magnesium_oxide#section=Top

Phase 7:

Rebuilding the WiFi Network

*Materials: **<u>Chemical-Free</u>** Foods and Cosmetics*

Tools: Plexus xFactor Plus™, Plexus® ProBio5, Plexus VitalBiome™, Plexus Bio Cleanse™, and Plexus Slim®

Chapter 12: Hormones and Hormone Disruptors

A WiFi network uses radio waves to send signals between devices across a network. These radio waves are often sent from a modem to computers, smartphones, home security systems, TVs, gaming systems, voice-activated speakers, lights, thermostats, and various other "smart" devices. Nowadays, WIFI controls a myriad of things, and in some respects, is what makes the home "operate."

Likewise, the temple of the body has its own sort of WIFI system called the endocrine system. The endocrine system is essentially the hormonal system. Hormones act like radio waves—little messengers that communicate with other parts of the body, similarly to the way a WIFI signal communicates with home devices.

Approximately 50 different hormones are sent from modem-like endocrine glands (the hypothalamus, pituitary gland, pancreas, ovaries, testes, thyroid, and adrenal glands, to name a few). They are transported via a network of fluids to rouse cells and tissue into action—but only cells that have those specific hormone receptors on them. The receptors are like the wireless card or wireless adaptor in a laptop. The laptop can't connect to WIFI without it. In the same way, cells can't use hormones without hormone receptors.

So, why are hormones so important? Well, because, like WIFI, they control a myriad of things in the temple. These messengers control almost all major bodily functions—from basic things like hunger and sleep to complex things like metabolism, reproduction, growth, development, and turning genes "on and off." They even control the stress response, emotions, and mood.

It's safe to say that the endocrine system impacts almost every organ, cell, and function of the body. So, when hormones are imbalanced, or the endocrine system is not working correctly, it can have an enormous domino effect in the body.

The endocrine system interacts with many other bodily systems. I have already mentioned many of them and their respective hormones in previous chapters. In this chapter, I will briefly recap some of those and relay a few more important points to consider.

However, please note: the endocrine system is very complex and intricate. This chapter is simply general information. Therefore, if you suspect you have hormone issues, it is imperative to see your doctor. Do NOT try to figure out hormone issues on your own. You absolutely must work with a licensed medical professional. Again, this chapter is just basic information as it relates to some hormones. I am not a doctor, and this information is not to replace medical advice.

Now, let's go over some of the main hormones in the temple. (Note: this is by no means a complete list.)

Blood Sugar Hormones

Insulin: As we discussed at the very beginning of this book, insulin is a hormone made in the pancreas that helps cells use glucose for energy. It helps maintain steady blood sugar levels. But it is also one of the most influential hormones in the body, so it is very closely linked to all other hormones, including testosterone and estrogen.

Glucagon: Glucagon is another hormone made in the pancreas that helps assist in the breakdown of glycogen (a form of glucose stored in the muscles and liver for the body's future energy needs). It releases this stored glucose to prevent blood sugar levels from dropping too low.

Stress Hormones

Cortisol: Cortisol is a stress hormone made by the adrenal glands. It regulates metabolism, salt/water balance, the immune system, and physical and emotional stress, among other things. During stressful moments, cortisol increases glucose in the bloodstream, so the body has enough energy to deal with the stress. It also helps the brain use glucose efficiently and helps the body repair tissue.

Adrenaline (A.K.A. epinephrine): Adrenaline is often called the "fight-or-flight" hormone. It increases heart rate, helps blood pump throughout the body, and helps oxygen get to muscles and the brain so the body can physically deal with the stress.

Thyroid Hormones

Thyroxine (T4): T4 is the primary thyroid hormone because the thyroid makes abundantly more of it than the other thyroid hormone, which is T3. However, some T4 is converted into T3 after it is released into the bloodstream.

Triiodothyronine (T3): T3 is the most "active" thyroid hormone. There is not as much of it produced by the thyroid, but it is said to have four times the strength of T4.

Thyroid hormones T4 and T3 are needed by every cell in the body for a healthy cellular metabolism. They also assist in maintaining blood pressure, muscle tone, heart rate, reproductive functions, digestion, among other things.

Sex Hormones

While sex hormones are categorized as male and female, it is important to note that it's normal for both men and women to have both estrogen and testosterone. It is the levels of these hormones that vary between the sexes.

Male Hormones: The testes produce androgen hormones such as testosterone. These hormones affect sexual development, facial hair/pubic hair, muscle mass, bone mass, libido, and sperm production.

Female Hormones: The ovaries produce estrogen and progesterone. The gut microbiome also produces active forms of estrogen (1) and metabolizes excess estrogen. (2) These hormones affect things such as breast growth, menstruation, pregnancy. Progesterone is important for implantation of a fertilized egg in the uterus and maintaining the pregnancy.

Symptoms of Hormone Imbalances

Hormone imbalances can cause many different and yet similar symptoms, depending on which hormones are imbalanced. Therefore, it is important to not only be aware of symptoms but also talk to your doctor about them. This is simply a general guideline, which can vary dramatically from person to person and symptom to symptom. Only a qualified licensed medical professional can diagnose hormone imbalances.

Symptoms of Imbalanced Blood Sugar Hormones

Having too much insulin can cause low blood sugar, which is known as hypoglycemia. Symptoms of hypoglycemia can include:

- Sweating
- Feeling clammy
- Chills

- Feeling lightheaded
- Dizziness
- Confusion
- Anxiety or nervousness
- Feeling shaky
- Increased heartbeat
- Hunger
- Irritability and impatience
- Blurred or double vision
- Tingling in the lips/mouth area

Not having enough insulin can cause high blood sugar, known as hyperglycemia. Symptoms of hyperglycemia can include:

- Increased thirst
- Blurred vision
- Weight loss
- Headaches
- Poor Concentration
- Frequent urination
- Fatigue

Because glucagon raises the blood sugar levels by releasing stored glucose, too much glucagon has the same symptoms as above (hyperglycemia), if it is not counteracted by insulin. Conversely, not having enough glucagon, can cause hypoglycemia and symptoms associated with that.

Symptoms of Imbalanced Stress Hormones

Having too much cortisol can result in symptoms such as:

- Anxiety and anxiety disorders
- Irritability
- Puffy face
- Insomnia
- Weight gain (especially in the face, upper back, and torso)
- Swelling (hands and feet)
- Thinning skin
- Stomach pain (especially in children)
- Easy bruising
- Erratic blood sugars
- Muscle weakness
- Acne
- Low libido

- Poor concentration or short-term memory
- Female balding

Having too little cortisol can result in symptoms such as:

- Loss of appetite
- Low blood pressure
- Salt cravings
- Nausea or vomiting
- Diarrhea
- Abdominal pain
- Darkened skin
- Muscle/ joint pain
- Fatigue (usually extreme)
- Irritability and/or depression
- Sexual dysfunction in women

Having too little adrenaline is extremely rare, but having too much adrenaline can result in symptoms such as:

- Fast heartbeat
- High blood pressure
- Anxiety
- Weight loss
- Excessive sweating

Symptoms of Imbalanced Thyroid Hormones

Having low levels of thyroid hormones is a condition known as hypothyroidism. Symptoms of hypothyroidism can include:

- Weight gain
- Swelling in the neck which could indicate a thyroid goiter
- Slower heartbeat
- Fatigue
- Hair loss
- Feeling cold
- Dry skin
- Brittle nails
- Numbness or tingling in the hands
- Constipation
- Abnormal menstrual periods

Having too high levels of thyroid hormones is a condition known as hyperthyroidism. Symptoms of hyperthyroidism can include:

- Weight loss
- Swelling in the neck
- Fast heartbeat
- Increased blood pressure
- Palpitations
- Restlessness, anxiety, and/or irritability
- Sleeping problems
- Hair loss
- Muscle weakness
- Trembling hands
- Vision problems
- Diarrhea
- Irregular menstrual periods

Symptoms of Imbalanced Estrogen in Women

Having too much estrogen in comparison to other sex hormones is often called "estrogen dominance." Symptoms of estrogen dominance in women can include:

- Bloating
- Trouble sleeping
- Fibrocystic breast lumps
- Increased symptoms of PMS
- Mood swings
- Headaches
- Anxiety and panic attacks
- Swelling and tenderness in breasts
- Weight gain (especially in hips, buttocks, and thighs, and occasionally in arms and breasts, too)
- Irregular menstrual periods
- Hair loss
- Low libido
- Cold hands or feet
- Fatigue
- Memory problems

Having too little estrogen in comparison to other sex hormones can cause women to have symptoms such as:

- Headaches and/or migraines
- Urinary tract infections

- Irregular or missed periods
- Mood swings
- Breast tenderness
- Depression
- Hot flashes
- Trouble concentrating
- Fatigue

Above symptoms could also indicate too little progesterone, as can heavy menstrual bleeding and gallbladder problems. Too much progesterone could cause the above symptoms as well as ovarian cysts.

Symptoms of Imbalanced Estrogen in Men

Having too little estrogen in comparison to other sex hormones can cause men to have symptoms such as:

- Fatigue
- Depression
- Joint cracking/pain
- Anxiety
- Unnecessary jealousy
- Low emotion
- Low orgasms
- Low blood pressure
- Excessive urination

Estrogen dominance can cause men to have symptoms such as:

- Increased abdominal fat
- Loss of muscle mass
- Low libido
- Erectile dysfunction
- Fatigue
- Increased fatty tissue around nipples
- Depression
- Emotional disturbances
- Urinary tract symptoms

Symptoms of Imbalanced Testosterone in Men

Having too much testosterone can cause men to have symptoms such as:

- Smaller testicles
- Lower sperm count

- Anger and/or Aggressiveness
- Impulsivity

Having too little testosterone can cause men to have symptoms such as:

- Low energy
- Reduced strength
- Decrease in stamina
- Aches/pains in the bones and joints
- Loss of libido
- Difficulty having erections
- Weight gain
- Osteoporosis

Symptoms of Imbalanced Testosterone in Women

Too much testosterone in women can cause symptoms such as:

- excess body / facial hair
- balding
- smaller breast size
- deeper voice
- acne
- increased muscle

Too little testosterone in women can cause symptoms such as:

- Decrease in libido
- Loss of motivation
- Less sexual satisfaction
- Depression
- Fatigue
- Muscle loss, weakness, or inability to maintain muscle
- Thinning skin

Investigating Problems

When problems arise with the WIFI in your home, it's not always obvious what is causing them. You often have to do some investigating to figure it out, usually with a professional because it could be any number of things.

It could be the signal strength—if you are too far away from the modem, the radio waves might not be able to reach the device. It could be the device itself—it might have a damaged access card that can't pick up the signal. It could be the modem—if it is damaged, it might not be able to send the signal. It could be the wiring on the modem—maybe there is a short in a cord or a broken connector. It could also be the WIFI source—perhaps the service has been interrupted because of an error with the service provider's tower or lines. Or perhaps the wiring to the home has been damaged, and the service is not getting from the lines to the modem. WIFI problems can be any number of things.

This is how it is with the temple WIFI system, also. When you suspect that you have "hormone problems" it's not always obvious what is causing them, and it can really be any number of things. Again, this is why you must call a professional to help get to the bottom of things.

Signal Strength

Sometimes hormone problems could be a problem with the "signal strength," where the hormones aren't making it to the target cells/tissue. After hormones are secreted from the gland they were produced in, many of them are bound to a "transport protein" that acts like a taxicab for the hormone. Transport proteins are made in the liver and basically "hold" hormones in their inactive state while they circulate the body looking for target cells to act in. Protein deficiency and liver problems can sometimes inhibit this transport to target cells.

Damage

Hormone issues could also be due to injury in the gland itself. Like a damaged modem, some hormone-producing organs could experience impairment too, which in turn affects hormone production and transmission. For example, certain autoimmune diseases can cause the immune system to accidentally attack its own tissue, like in the case of Grave's Disease or Hashimoto's Disease, where it attacks the thyroid gland. Other glandular factors could also include injury to the testes, ovarian cysts, and head trauma affecting the hypothalamus and/or pituitary gland.

Outside Sources/Precursors

Hormone issues could also be related to external sources. Like radio waves that originate outside the house, hormones can also come from things outside the actual hormone-producing organ. Some hormones like cortisol, DHEA, testosterone, estrogen, and progesterone derive from cholesterol. Other hormones like thyroid hormones, serotonin, epinephrine, norepinephrine, histamine, and melatonin derive from amino acids, which are the building blocks of proteins. And eicosanoids (which assist with things like blood vessel constriction and inflammation) derive from polyunsaturated fat.

In addition to that, vitamins and minerals are often needed to make and use hormones. For example, vitamin B5 is used to make both sex hormones and stress hormones. Iodine is needed for the thyroid to produce T4 and T3. Selenium is needed to convert T4 into T3 (without selenium there can be no activation of thyroid hormones). And boron is needed to use estrogen and testosterone. (3) (4) These are just a few examples that illustrate how important a nutritionally sound diet is for a well-functioning endocrine system and hormone balance.

The Seesaw and the Web

When investigating hormone issues with your doctor, it's important to be honest about all your symptoms, even if they seem unrelated, because these "seemingly unrelated things" could point to hormone _imbalance_.

The hormones circulating throughout the body should maintain a very precise equilibrium. It's not that there should be the same amount or the same level of each hormone in the body. But instead, each hormone should be produced at and circulate at 100% of its unique level needed by the body. When there is 100% (or "enough") of each hormone circulating the body (and active), that is called hormone balance. When there is not enough of one or an overabundance of another, that is imbalanced.

This goes for "types" of hormones too. The types of hormones should balance each other, like a 4-way see-saw at the playground. If each child weighs the same, the seesaw stays in balance. But if you put a small toddler in one seat, two medium-sized children in two other seats, and a large teenager in the 4th seat, the see-saw will not be balanced. This is like the endocrine scale.

Hormones try to compensate for each other. If one hormone is lacking, another hormone might go into overdrive to make up for it. That imbalance can then lead to another imbalance, and then another, creating a sort of domino effect of imbalance. Put simply; nearly all hormones affect each other in some way.

The stress hormone, cortisol, is one example. It's like the large teenager on the see-saw, affecting almost everything! Cortisol is insulin's counterpart. It takes sugar stored in the liver (glycogen) and puts it into the bloodstream. So too much cortisol can substantially raise blood sugar levels, which then can increase insulin, and slow metabolism by affecting the thyroid.

Another example: estrogen is carried by a transport protein called "sex hormone-binding globulin." However, too much of this is associated with a less active thyroid hormone. Low estrogen can also hinder insulin production in the pancreas and impair the action of insulin in the cells. In fact, a decrease in estrogen has been found to increase insulin resistance in both men and women. (5)

Therefore, when investigating hormones, it's important to consult a doctor like an endocrinologist who is qualified enough to look at the whole person—the "big picture." It may not be just one hormone, or even one type of hormone, that is out of whack. Not only that, the endocrine system is like a huge, comprehensive spider web, interconnected with itself and other systems, so sometimes multiple glands and precursors can be involved also.

For example, let's look at "thyroid problems." The hypothalamus tells the pituitary gland to produce what's called a "Thyroid Stimulating Hormone" (TSH), which tells the thyroid to make thyroid hormones. But, in order to make them, the thyroid takes iodine from food and combines it with the amino acid tyrosine (also from food), then it uses these to make T4. The body then uses selenium to convert the T4 to T3.

So, if you have a "thyroid problem," the question becomes: where did the problem originate? Is it a problem in the hypothalamus, pituitary gland, the thyroid gland itself, or in the conversion process because of an iodine, selenium or tyrosine deficiency? Or, is it an autoimmune issue, related to gluten or dairy intolerance or allergy? (Remember, gluten and dairy proteins resemble the thyroid gland, and sometimes immune cells attack the thyroid by mistake, thinking it is gluten or dairy.) So, you will want to work with a doctor who will take all of these factors into consideration. Testing just TSH and T4 levels is often not enough.

The same is true for imbalances with sex hormones. For example, the pituitary gland sends FSH and LH that tell the ovaries to make progesterone and estrogen (it tells the testicles to make testosterone too). But all three forms of estrogen can also be re-activated in the gut as well. So again, if you have an "estrogen imbalance" where does the imbalance come from? Is it related to a gut issue like SIBO or Candida? Is it a problem with the ovaries themselves? Is there not an adequate supply of cholesterol or vitamin B5 to make estrogen? Or, is it a problem originating in the pituitary gland in the brain because of things like heavy metal toxicity? Again, there are multiple layers to consider, so it is important to work with a doctor who is willing to look at all possibilities.

The Top Ten Things That Might Be Messing with Your Hormones

There are so many various things that can affect hormones, that it's impossible to cover them all. However, there are ten things that can be huge contributors. Talk to your doctor to determine if these may be having an impact on you.

1. *Natural Causes*

Sometimes imbalances are not a result of damage or dysfunction per se, but instead natural factors, such as aging. This takes place in both men and women. For example, women start with a balanced progesterone/estrogen ratio. Then, during a women's 30s progesterone begins to decline, sometimes rapidly. Estrogen levels drop too, but not as sharp as progesterone. This can lead to what is known as estrogen dominance...where the estrogen-progesterone ratio becomes skewed because of declining progesterone. Symptoms of estrogen dominance might include mood swings, irritability, anxiety, bloating, weight gain, skin issues, and irregular or heavier periods.

In a woman's 40s and 50s estrogen levels become more erratic during perimenopause and menopause. Estrogen begins to drop more dramatically like progesterone did, but it does not drop steadily. These ups and downs can cause symptoms such as mood swings, hot flashes, and night sweats. But, eventually, estrogen drops low enough to reach progesterone again, and they come back into balance.

In men, testosterone levels reach their peak around 17 or 18 years old, but it can start to decrease around age 40. Unlike a woman's "drop" in hormones, though, a man's is more gradual. Testosterone decreases slowly and steadily, approximately 1% each year. This might seem insignificant, but after two or three decades, it equates to 20-30% less testosterone production than peak years.

Hormone Disruptors:

Additionally, there are also chemicals and toxins in food and the environment that are known "endocrine or hormone disruptors." This means these substances disrupt hormone signaling in the body for both men and women. Some endocrine disruptors *impersonate* hormones. They act like identity thieves, binding to hormone receptors, and sending out false signals. Others hormone disruptors prevent hormones from binding to the receptors altogether. And some hormone disruptors can change how much of a hormone is made, even the way it behaves in cells. In my opinion, the most common and often the most detrimental hormone disruptors are:

2.   *PCBs*

PCBs are chemicals technically called polychlorinated biphenyls. They were once used in making electric material, capacitors, transformers, and in heat transfer fluids. They are no longer used in the United States today, but they can still be found in some landfills containing these older products. PCBs can also evaporate from contaminated water, such as the Great Lakes. They interfere mostly with thyroid hormones (6) by disrupting both the production and distribution of T4 and T3. (7)

3. *Dioxins:*

Dioxins are a group of about 219 highly toxic chlorinated compounds that are produced during manufacturing processes like herbicide production and paper bleaching. They are emitted into the air from these factories and then enter the water, soil, and plants nearby. Surrounding farms then become contaminated as do animals and fish. Dioxins accumulate in the fat tissue of these animals and fish and then accumulate in the fat tissue of the humans who consume them. Cattle that have significant fat tissue amass the most, and so beef and dairy products often contain the highest levels of dioxins. (8)

Additionally, the EPA estimates 40% of dioxins from bleached coffee filters transfer to your coffee. Dioxins are also in the pesticide and herbicide residue on non-organic produce, as well as in chlorine bleach and triclosan. Triclosan is a germ fighter that can turn into dioxin in sunlight. It is added to antibacterial soaps, deodorants, toothpaste, even some water sources.

Dioxins stimulate estrogen receptor signaling and negatively affect the body's response to hormones. (9) It's also been found that dioxins decrease estradiol (a form of estrogen) secretion as well as progesterone and steroid hormones. (10)

4. *Xenoestrogens:*

Xenoestrogens are synthetic or sometimes even natural compounds that mimic estrogen and can lead to estrogen dominance (having too much estrogen). Xeno means "foreign," so these are things that are not normally present in the body.

Research has found that there are approximately 31 legal food additives (such as Propyl gallate and 4-Hexylresorcinol) that can potentially mimic estrogen. (11) These are found in things like candy, processed meat, throat lozenges, dried milk, baked goods, mouthwash, sunscreen, and herbicides such as glyphosate (31) to name only a few.

5. *Soy:*

Not only do non-organic soybeans contain glyphosate, but soy in general (organic or non-organic) contains active ingredients known as isoflavones which are structurally similar to estrogen. They are natural xenoestrogens because they can initiate a response from estrogen receptors (and can also interfere with steroid metabolism).

Some claim that isoflavones in soy can be helpful during menopause when estrogen levels drop. However, I advise using caution, as there is far more to consider. One, if it is not organic or non-GMO soy, it could contain extremely high levels of harmful pesticides. (12) Two, estrogen stimulates breast cancer cells helping them grow and spread. (13) So, if you have a family history of estrogenic cancers (breast, endometrial, colorectal, or uterine), if you started menstruation early, or started menopause late, you may want to talk to your doctor about this, and seriously consider reducing your soy and xenoestrogen exposure. (14)

And this goes for men too. Even though it is often just associated with women, men have estrogen also and can experience hormone imbalances too. Having too much estrogen can skew a man's estrogen/testosterone ratio leading to symptoms such as depression, low libido, erectile dysfunction, enlarged breasts (sometimes referred to as "man boobs"), decreased muscle mass, and fatigue. Studies show that soy isoflavones can affect free testosterone levels in men (15) and are associated with low sperm count. (16) So, men should also be mindful of their exposure to xenoestrogens and other hormone disruptors.

Other factors that can also affect testosterone levels are age, alcohol (too much alcohol can interrupt the signaling from the brain to the testicles), liver problems (17), and lack of sleep. In fact, one study found that a loss of sleep can drastically lower testosterone levels in just one week. Some levels even dropped by 10-15%! (18)

6. *Conventional Beef and Dairy Products*

Dairy and cattle farmers often give cows hormones to increase milk supply or fatten them before slaughter. These hormones end up in the meat and the milk of the animal, which then can be transferred to the humans who consumes them. Also, naturally occurring hormones can be transferred to humans as well.

Some of the hormones that have been found in cow's milk and other dairy products are prolactin, estrogens, progesterone, corticoids, androgens, insulin-like growth factor-1 (IGF-1), and prostaglandins. (19) Because hormones like estrogen are fat-soluble, whole milk likely contains more than skim milk. Conventional beef has also been found to contain hormones, even naturally occurring estrogen. (20)

7. *Wheat and Other Grains:*

There is a type of fungus called zearalenone that colonizes on barley, corn, wheat, and other grains. It, too, is similar to estrogen and has been said to contribute to congenital disabilities in grain-fed farm animals, early breast development in young girls, and the reduced effectiveness of two drugs used for breast cancer treatment. (21)

8. *Parabens:*

Parabens are synthetic chemicals found in pharmaceuticals, foods, and cosmetics. The most common are methylparaben, ethylparaben, propylparaben, isobutylparaben, butylparaben, and benzylparaben... basically anything that ends in "paraben." What makes parabens problematic is that parabens have estrogen-like properties. They act like synthetic estrogen in the body. In fact, they have even been known to cause breast cells (both normal and cancerous) to grow and divide. In fact, actual parabens have been found in breast cancer tissue – in tumors! And not just in a few cases. They were present in 99% of those who were studied! (22) (23)

9. *Plastics:*

You have probably heard it before, that plastic products contain chemicals (like BPA) that act like estrogen in the body. Maybe you've even started looking for BPA-free water bottles and cups. But it's not just BPA that is harmful. Studies show that almost ALL plastic products (regardless of the type of resin, product, or retail source) leach chemicals with estrogenic activity—including those advertised as BPA free! In fact, in some cases, the BPA-free products released chemicals with more estrogenic activity than the BPA-containing products! (24) It may be worth getting rid of all plastic dishes in your kitchen, and start using glass.

10. *Statins and other drugs*

Recently, many clinicians have come forth to express their concerns about the impact of cholesterol-reducing drugs, which includes how they affect hormone balance. (25) As I mentioned before, cholesterol is crucial for hormone production. And statins have been found to lower hormones in both men and women (26) The overuse or long-term use of prescription corticosteroid medications (including corticosteroid injections) can increase cortisol levels—and remember, cortisol is the teenager on the seesaw, and can potentially affect other hormones. If you are currently taking these medications, and are concerned about hormone balance, it is important to discuss these concerns with your doctor.

Also, it's important to note that illegal drugs such as marijuana contain phytoestrogens that can interfere with normal hormone signaling. (27) And, the THC compounds in marijuana also raise cortisol (the stress hormone), lower prolactin (the sex-gratification hormone) (28), disrupt menstrual cycle and inhibit the release of eggs from ovaries (29), provoke early puberty and stunt growth in boys (30), and alter sperm and affect fertility. (31)

Again (I cannot stress this enough), the endocrine system is enormously complex. If you suspect you have hormone issues, it is very important to work closely with an experienced doctor who can investigate possible root causes by doing comprehensive lab work and talking to you about your diet, your lifestyle, and other related factors, leaving no stone unturned.

But do not get overwhelmed with this list. Your challenge today is to pick just one hormone-disrupting thing and eliminate it from your life ASAP (except medications, do not get rid of those without your doctor's consent). Pick just one. Maybe start buying organic beef or get rid of all the plastic in your kitchen. Then, when that has become your "new norm," pick something else on the list. Maybe start looking at beauty products or reading labels.

Below is a list created by Rachael Pontillo of several xenoestrogen producing chemicals. Again, don't let this overwhelm you. Take it slow. There is no time table on how fast you have to absorb this information. Pick a few and memorize them. Then in a few days or weeks, memorize a few more. Or, better yet, don't use or eat anything you can't pronounce.

Chemicals That Could Interfere with Hormone Balance:

1. Ethinylestradiol (oral contraceptive pill)
2. Propyl gallate
3. Alkylphenol
4. Phthalates
5. 4-Methylbenzylidene camphor (4-MBC)
6. Phenosulfothiazine
7. Erythrosine / FD&C Red No. 3
8. Heptachlor
9. Lindane /hexachlorocyclohexane
10. Chlorine
11. Dichlorodiphenyldichloroethylene
12. Metalloestrogens
13. Butylated hydroxyanisole / BHA
14. Methoxychlor
15. Endosulfan
16. Atrazine
17. Nonylphenol and derivatives
18. Dieldrin
19. Pentachlorophenol
20. DDT
21. Polychlorinated biphenyls / PCBs
22. Parabens
23. DEHP

References:

(1) https://www.ncbi.nlm.nih.gov/pubmed/28778332

(2) https://www.ncbi.nlm.nih.gov/pubmed/27107051

(3) https://www.ncbi.nlm.nih.gov/pmc/articles/PMC4712861/

(4) https://www.ncbi.nlm.nih.gov/pmc/articles/PMC1566640/

(5) https://www.ncbi.nlm.nih.gov/pubmed/21984197

(6) https://www.ncbi.nlm.nih.gov/pmc/articles/PMC1257681/

(7) http://enhs.umn.edu/current/5103/endocrine/mechanisms.html

(8) https://www.aphis.usda.gov/animal_health/emergingissues/downloads/dioxins.pdf

(9) https://www.the-scientist.com/?articles.view/articleNo/22212/title/Dioxins--estrogen-connection/

(10) http://www.scielo.br/scielo.php?script=sci_arttext&pid=S0102-311X2002000200010

(11) https://www.ncbi.nlm.nih.gov/pubmed?orig_db=PubMed&cmd=Search&TransSchema=title&term=%22Chemical+research+in+toxicology%22%5BJour%5D+AND+Identification+of+Xenoestrogens+

(12) https://www.sciencedirect.com/science/article/pii/S0308814613019201

(13) https://www.cancer.org/cancer/breast-cancer/treatment/hormone-therapy-for-breast-cancer.html

(14) https://www.ncbi.nlm.nih.gov/pubmed/17113977

(15) https://www.ncbi.nlm.nih.gov/pubmed/21353476

(16) https://www.ncbi.nlm.nih.gov/pubmed/18650557

(17) https://www.ncbi.nlm.nih.gov/pubmed/25087838

(18) https://www.ncbi.nlm.nih.gov/pmc/articles/PMC4445839/

(19) https://www.ncbi.nlm.nih.gov/pmc/articles/PMC4524299/

(20) https://www.sciencedirect.com/science/article/pii/S1021949816300394#bib10

(21) http://www.newswise.com/articles/estrogen-mimicking-compounds-in-foods-may-reduce-effectiveness-of-breast-cancer-treatment

(22) https://www.ncbi.nlm.nih.gov/pubmed/14745841

(23) https://www.huffingtonpost.com/organic-authoritycom/breast-cancer-parabens-b_1209041.html

(24) https://www.ncbi.nlm.nih.gov/pmc/articles/PMC3222987/

(25) https://www.huffingtonpost.com/kelly-brogan-md/women-statins_b_4283650.html

(26) https://bmcmedicine.biomedcentral.com/articles/10.1186/1741-7015-11-57

(27) https://www.ncbi.nlm.nih.gov/pubmed/6296360

(28) https://www.ncbi.nlm.nih.gov/pubmed/22885247

(29) https://www.ncbi.nlm.nih.gov/pmc/articles/PMC4918871/

(30) https://www.sciencedaily.com/releases/2015/05/150518191604.htm

(31) https://www.parenting.com/fertility/infertility/smoking-marijuana-may-morph-sperm-affect-fertility

(32) https://www.ncbi.nlm.nih.gov/pubmed/23756170

Chapter 13: Big, Bad Stress Hormones

While all hormones are important when rebuilding your temple—and keeping a balanced "seesaw"—I'd like to spend a little more time talking about the big, bad teenager on the seesaw, aka stress hormones.

When your brain detects a threat, like say an intruder in your house, neurotransmitters like dopamine and norepinephrine are released. These activate the amygdala area of the brain, which triggers an emotional response to the stress—for example, fear. These also signal the hippocampus in the brain to store the emotional experience in long-term memory.

The threat also triggers the release of stress hormones such as adrenaline and cortisol. This is a good thing. It's your body's way of preparing for the threat, and it is often referred to as the "fight or flight" response.

Adrenaline gives you the "boost" you need. It raises the heart rate, increases blood flow to the muscles, increases blood output from the heart, dilates pupils, etc. It gears you up, so to speak. Cortisol puts all non-essential body functions (like immune and digestive functions) on hold, so the body can focus all its energy on dealing with the threat. And because the body needs *immediate* energy to deal with the situation, cortisol quickly raises blood sugar. It tells glucagon to release the stored glucose from the liver, and it tells insulin to stop storing glucose so it will be available as immediate energy during the stress. Once the threat is over, cortisol signals the body to eat and replenish the glucose that was lost.

Sounds like an efficient process, right? Well, not always. The problem is, this "fight or flight" response happens with any type of perceived stress—even if it's not *physical* stress as in the case of an intruder. This response can happen when we are "threatened" with a work deadline, an unpaid bill, or a verbally abusive relationship. In these instances, stress hormones are released, and the body gears up for battle, but no *physical* "battle" ever takes place.

Adrenaline increases heart rate, and cortisol increases glucose, but the body doesn't burn all that fuel because there's no fight, and there's no flight. Regardless, cortisol still signals the body to eat again, though, to replenish what *should* be lost glucose (this is where "stress eating" comes from).

The other problem is that this stress response is supposed to be a *temporary* response, enabling the body to deal with a *momentary* threat. Stresses such as unpaid bills and unhealthy relationships don't typically resolve quickly, and so the body can remain in "fight or flight" longer than it is supposed to.

And as you can imagine, prolonged periods of increased heart rate and suppressed immune and digestive function are not ideal. Studies have also connected long-term exposure to cortisol to a shrinking of the hippocampus, the brain's memory center. It is not known yet whether this shrinking is reversible. (1)

What's more, this chronic stress can increase intestinal permeability, a.k.a. leaky gut (2), cause insulin resistance (3), decrease bone formation, decrease memory, and lead to widespread inflammation and pain. (4) It can also cause adrenal fatigue, where the adrenal glands become weakened (fatigued) from overuse, and no longer know how to efficiently respond to stress. (Some doctors don't recognize this as a medical diagnosis yet, but it's worth mentioning because I've known many people with adrenal fatigue symptoms.)

Also, because adrenaline raises heart rate and dramatically increases blood flow, chronic stress can contribute to long-term heart and blood vessel problems, as well as inflammation in the circulatory system, especially in the coronary arteries. These effects are sometimes worse for post-menopausal women with lower estrogen because estrogen helps blood vessels respond to stress. (5) Because the sympathetic nervous system (SNS) is what signals the adrenal glands to release adrenalin and cortisol, long term stress can cause wear and tear on the SNS too, which can, in turn, affect the reproductive systems in both men and women.

If that wasn't bad enough, long-term cortisol exposure can lead to an increase in belly fat, known as visceral fat. (6) (7) Visceral fat is different from subcutaneous fat which is located near the skin. Subcutaneous fat is the "pinch an inch" fat on love handles that you can grab with your fingers. Visceral fat, on the other hand, is a dangerous kind of fat located deeper in the abdomen, that surrounds vital organs. It's not relative to obesity either since it's just in the abdomen and not on thighs, buttocks, or anywhere else. This is why some people have potbellies but are otherwise skinny everywhere else. Generally, a waist size of 35 inches or more for women, and 40 inches or more for men, is an indicator of visceral fat.

What makes this so problematic is that visceral fat acts like an endocrine organ and secretes hormones and other chemicals linked to disease. In fact, research has shown a direct link between waist circumference and coronary heart disease (8), dementia (9), and cancer. In fact, premenopausal women whose waists are nearly as big as their hips have a three- to four-times higher risk of getting breast cancer than normal-weight women. (10)

What's more, belly fat has an abundant supply of cortisol receptors that bind the cortisol with fat. (11) It also has enzymes that convert inactive cortisone to active cortisol. So, visceral fat not only attracts cortisol; it activates it.

To make matters worse, cortisol can mobilize triglycerides that are in storage and relocate them to the abdomen. Yes, you read that right. Cortisol can basically take fat from your butt and move it to your belly. This creates a vicious cycle that looks something like this: stress increases cortisol > which increases belly fat >which further increases cortisol, which further increases belly fat, and so forth and so on.

Change the Changeable

Plain and simple: in order to break the cycle that is causing excess cortisol (the big teenager ruining the seesaw balance), we have to do something about stress.

First and foremost, consider talking to a professional (a licensed therapist), especially if the stress is chronic and now affecting your health. Next, work with a therapist, counselor, or certified life coach who can help you change the changeable. For example, if you are chronically stressed because you have too much on your plate, it might be time to adjust your schedule or lighten your load. Take a good, hard look at your daily responsibilities and see if there are things you can get rid of, at least for the time being.

This is hard, I know because these things are on your plate for a reason. They are all important to you to some degree or another—or you wouldn't be sabotaging your health trying to keep up with it all. But the cold hard unavoidable truth is: not everything we do is _equally_ important, and only YOU can order these things appropriately.

Occasionally, I have had clients tell me that there is nothing that can be put aside. They are just "too busy," too in demand, and so they want a "plan B." I think, for some people, their busyness makes them feel needed and productive, and so their ego is not yet willing to hand off tasks to other people. They cling to their full schedule like a security blanket... but, in reality, it's more like clinging to a grenade.

Unfortunately, there is no "plan B" for being too busy. If you have chronic stress because you are overburdened, and it is now affecting your health, then YOU have to adjust your workload. Well, I guess you don't "have" to. You can continue as you are, but given the numerous body systems affected by chronic stress, it hardly seems worth it to me.

In my opinion, the best way to determine which things you can get rid of is to prioritize them by number. This makes it easier to see that not everything is equal, and it makes it easier to say "no" to the things that fall low on the list.

This brings up another crucial point: saying no. It is not a crime to say no to someone who needs something. It does not make you a bad friend, a bad parent, a bad sibling, or a bad coworker... if you are genuinely and sincerely trying to order your life and get healthy. And, just because they asked you, doesn't mean you are the only person on the planet capable of assisting them. (Although, if you truly are the only person on the planet that can help, then perhaps you just need to get rid of a few other lower-ranked duties to make time for it.)

The point is: not everything is "necessary." For example, if your son or daughter wants to join ANOTHER extra-curricular activity this fall, or go to another party, or another sleepover.... and it will not only add substantially to your weekly drive time but also take away from family dinner and your own personal downtime, then perhaps it is not "necessary." Maybe you should say no. The child may be disappointed, yes, but I'm fairly certain he or she will not die without the activity. There have been many times where my husband and I have told our children no, simply for the sake of our own peace and sanity. And I have absolutely no regrets.

Relationships

Sometimes there are things that are little trickier than a schedule. Sometimes we are involved in toxic relationships that include constant manipulation, condemnation, and/or deceit. Sometimes it even involves mental, emotional, and/or physical abuse. These types of ongoing situations can have a dramatic effect on our stress response system and may require assistance from a mental or behavioral health professional who can help you navigate through this.

While it is rare that we can change the actual person causing the abuse, we *can* sometimes change our exposure to them. Sometimes, the best and most effective way to do this is to distance yourself from the person. If it is an acquaintance, family member, or friend who does not live in your home, you can start by screening your texts and calls, staying off social media, and avoiding the social events you know they will be at.

You do not need to be confrontational to do this. You can simply keep your distance. If they ask you about the distance, you can inform them that you need time to yourself to get healthy and work through some things.

215

If the person is violent, does not respect your request, or is currently inescapable because he/she lives in your home, you may need the assistance of law enforcement, a qualified social worker, or another professional who can advise you how to deal with this person safely. Sometimes, a protection from abuse (PFA) order may even be necessary. If the person is inescapable because he/she is your boss or coworker, it may be wise to consider looking for a new job, if it is clearly affecting your health and there is no way to distance yourself from that person.

Coping with the Unchangeable

Trauma

Sometimes, there are things that happen to us, like a trauma, that are unchangeable. We can't prevent it from happening, and we can't undo it after it has happened. The problem is, just one traumatic event can lead to *chronic* symptoms because traumatic experiences can embed in the memory of a person and arouse a stress response at any point, even when the person is no longer in danger. The person essentially relives the trauma through sporadic, unwilled flashbacks and nightmares, that they cannot control. He or she reexperiences the severe fight or flight response over and over again, and this memory can have the same physically-damaging effects as the real danger. This is called posttraumatic stress disorder (PTSD), and it is especially damaging if the trauma is repeated and chronic, like in the case of military combat or abuse.

It is even more severe in cases of childhood trauma because the child's brain is still forming and developing. Studies have shown that early, childhood stress can have a lasting effect on the HPA (hypothalamus-pituitary-adrenal) axis and norepinephrine. (12) In fact, trauma changes the biology of a child to such a degree that it can even be passed down to the next generation via epigenetic "intergenerational transmission." Children then of traumatized parents are at risk for similar stress-related problems (13), especially if they then are exposed to trauma as well.

It's also important to remember that stress is perception-based. The entire stress response system begins when the brain "perceives" a threat. That means something that may not be stressful for one person could be *highly* stressful for another person—especially if that person has been predisposed to stress dysfunction because of genetics, trauma, or even a parent's stress. (Young children of mothers who are highly stressed tend to be at high-risk for developing stress-related problems later on.) (1)

So, for these people, little stressors can be big stressors. For the most part, this is unchangeable for them. They are what I call "stress-sensitive." So, telling them to "calm down" is not effective because the stress response is beyond their control.

There are also many other types of on-going stressors that are often unavoidable and beyond one's control—losing a loved one, caring for someone who is chronically ill, living in poverty, experiencing an injury, being a single parent, and losing your job, to name a few.

In these cases, what can be done about the big teenager on the seesaw? Well, if you can't change the situation, try to manage the reaction. Below are what I consider to be the most important coping strategies for managing the stress response. But again, I am not a doctor or licensed counselor, so it is imperative to discuss your stress with a professional.

Therapy/Counseling

When rebuilding your stress response system, a mental health professional should serve as the foreman of the project, sometimes in conjunction with an endocrinologist. This is crucial if you are experiencing unmanageable acute stress or chronic stress (especially if it involves anxiety or depression). A licensed therapist or counselor can help you implement invaluable coping strategies and evaluate whether the stress is severe enough to warrant medication. I realize for some people, seeing a therapist has a stigma attached to it, but I think this is only because therapy is such a private subject that is not often talked about. The reality is, 42% of American adults have seen a counselor at some point in their lives. (14) I personally am one of them and have benefitted greatly from it. In fact, this is a massive understatement.

Exercise

Exercise is another great way to manage stress because it can serve as the missing "fight or flight" component in emotional or mental stress, burning up cortisol, and using extra glucose. However, not all types of exercise have the same effect. Studies have shown that moderate to high-intensity exercise *increases* cortisol levels, whereas low-intensity exercise reduces it. (15) Be sure to talk to your doctor about which type of exercise is safe for you.

If you are already suffering from stress dysfunction and high cortisol levels, it might be better to adopt low-intensity aerobic activities like walking and jogging versus an extreme exercise regimen like marathon training. Even high-intensity interval training can be problematic for the stress response system if you are overtraining. Overtraining can also result in cellular damage and hyperactivity of the immune system, which can contribute to the development of autoimmune conditions (16) as well as HPA axis dysfunction.

If you are chronically stressed, you may want to consider just doing approximately 30 minutes of daily aerobic activity. Or at the very least, mix up your regimen. Rotate low-intensity activity with high-intensity activity so that you do not risk overtraining.

As you condition yourself to handle exercise, you can simultaneously condition your stress response system too. Exercise releases cortisol and then naturally brings it back down to normal levels. Regular exercise can "retrain" the body so that when cortisol rises because of stress, it lowers more easily because it has been primed to do so during exercise. Again, consult your doctor before jumping into an exercise regimen with chronic stress.

Prayer and Mindfulness

Some of you may be wondering what the heck prayer and mindfulness have to do with rebuilding the stress response system. Let me just say it has *a lot* to do with it. The basis of both is silence. Finding silence removes us from the chaos, the noise, the stress... it pulls the mind (which controls the stress response) away from the hamster-wheel of worry so that we can just sit.

Sit how? As a Christian, I sit in prayer. There are many forms of prayer (Scripture reading, journaling, recitation, meditation, worship, to name a few). But what makes them important in terms of stress management is that they can invoke mindfulness.

Mindfulness is the process of becoming fully aware of the present moment. In the present moment, you're not focused on the past—the injustices or regret. You're not focused on the future—the fears or uncertainty. You're just focused on the here and now. And the Christian belief is that you are not alone in the "here and now." Instead, God is with you in it—caring for you, calling you, guiding you, providing for you. The Christian belief calls to mind that we are loved, forgiven, endowed with purpose, and destined for happiness. Being fully-mindful of this can have an enormous impact on stress.

And this is not just my "belief." Various mental health organizations are now employing these and other mindfulness-based stress reduction (MBSR) techniques or mindfulness-based cognitive therapies (MBCT) as part of their practice. Studies have shown that MBSR methods reduce cortisol levels (17) and are beneficial for those with social anxiety disorder. (18) Other studies showed that MBCT reduced depression by 57%, the recurrence rate of depression by 40–50%, anxiety levels by 58%, and stress levels by 40%. (19) Mindfulness has also been found to boost working memory, increase focus, improve relationship satisfaction, enhance fear modulation, improve immune function, and decrease emotional reactivity. (20)

Food for Cortisol Balance

One of the jobs of cortisol is to regulate the body's 24-hour rhythm (known as the circadian rhythm); therefore, cortisol levels fluctuate throughout the day. As mentioned earlier, you should have more energy (and therefore more cortisol) in the morning to get you out of bed. You should have less energy (and less cortisol) in the evening, to enjoy restful sleep. Typically, cortisol levels are highest around 7 a.m. and lowest around 3 a.m. with a sharp cortisol increase (up to 50%) twenty to thirty minutes after you wake up.

When cortisol levels are dysregulated, though, you may notice an alertness or a "second wind" in the evening because cortisol levels are high when they should be low. Or you may notice you wake up too early (even in the middle of the night) and are not able to get back to sleep because again, cortisol levels are high when they should be low. You may also notice that you are exhausted in the morning and can't ever seem to "get going," likely because cortisol levels are low when they should be high.

In these cases, food is either your best friend or your worst enemy. When and what you eat can either help bring cortisol back into balance or make matters worse.

As I mentioned before, the release of cortisol causes blood sugar levels to rise (for energy). Eating a high carb breakfast then (when glucose is already high), can raise them even higher and cause a surge of insulin, which can potentially drop them too low. This can set the stage for a day full of erratic blood sugars, fatigue, cravings, and more stress.

This is why some (myself included) say that breakfast is the most important meal of the day. It can make or break the rest of your day. If you have high or dysregulated cortisol, it's essential to eat protein and fat at breakfast. I want to challenge you to start thinking of breakfast differently. It doesn't have to be high carb cereals, bagels, and pastries like we're conditioned to see on television commercials. Instead, one of the best (and my personal favorite) breakfast options is keto dinner leftovers. When I eat dinner leftovers for breakfast I notice my blood sugars, stress response, and appetite are all more balanced throughout the day. When I eat a high carb breakfast (especially high carb, high sugar), I typically have more cravings and am more easily aggravated. I also tend to have more brain fog, too.

Social Connections

Lack of social interaction can also increase anxiety. In fact, it's been found that loneliness raises stress hormones and blood pressure. It undermines regulation of the circulatory system so that the heart muscle works harder, and the blood vessels are subject to damage. (21) This is important nowadays when so many interactions take place via social media and texting rather than face-to-face, in person. Studies are showing a direct correlation between the time spent on social media and feelings of perceived social isolation. (22)

Reduce Trigger Foods

Breakfast is not the only meal to be careful with if you're trying to lower cortisol. You should be mindful at *every* meal, avoiding trigger foods that can potentially raise stress hormones. The most common are: dairy, sugar, gluten, soy, fruit juice, alcohol, and caffeine. As a rule of thumb, all foods with a high glycemic index (GI) rating can increase cortisol.

Tools to Help Cope with Stress and Mood

In addition to lifestyle changes and coping strategies, there are multiple tools that may be beneficial when attempting to rebuild your stress response system. These are what I consider to be the most valuable tools in my personal toolbelt. Ask your doctor if they are safe for you.

Prebiotics and Probiotics

We've already talked extensively about the gut-brain connection, but it's important to reiterate it here because the gut microbiome affects the stress response system too. In fact, it's been found that even short-term exposure to stress can impact the microbiome by altering amounts of the main bacteria's phyla (its major "lineages"). And this can become a vicious cycle because alterations can then affect stress responsiveness, anxiety-like behavior, and the setpoint for activation of HPA axis. (23)

For this reason, it can be quite beneficial to start incorporating probiotics and prebiotics into the daily regimen. Research has shown that probiotics can substantially lower blood cortisol levels (24), and prebiotic intake can reduce waking cortisol, as well as alter emotions. (25)

In regards to prebiotics, I personally take the Plexus Slim® and Plexus Lean™. As I have already mentioned in earlier phases, Slim and Lean contain prebiotics that have been clinically proven to feed good microbes.

Regarding probiotics, I take both Plexus® ProBio5 and Plexus VitalBiome™ as well. As I already mentioned, VitalBiome™ contains eight strains of good bacteria that are specifically relevant to stress (Lactobacillus Helveticus, Bifidobacterium

Longum, Bacillus Coagulans, Lactobacillus Acidophilus, Lactobacillus Plantarum, Bifidobacterium Lactis, and Bifidobacterium Lactis).

For example, the Lactobacillus and Bifidobacterium families of bacteria are often considered "psychobiotics" because they can produce positive psychiatric effects when taken in appropriate quantities. The impact of psychobiotics falls into three categories: effects on emotional and cognitive processes, effects on the HPA axis and cortisol response, and effects on neurotransmitters and proteins. (26)

Lactobacillus Plantarum is psychobiotic because it falls into two of the three categories. It's been shown to reduce cortisol levels in human saliva (27), and increase dopamine and serotonin levels in mice, even with psychotropic effects. (28) Bifidobacterium Longum is psychobiotic because it, too, falls into two of the three categories. It's been found to reduce cortisol and enhance memory and frontal mobility. (29)

Vitamins

As I mentioned earlier, Plexus xFactor Plus™ is a "microbiome activating" complex which can be beneficial in stress management, but it also contains 100% (or more) of the Daily Value of nineteen essential vitamins and minerals and over 50 naturally occurring trace minerals. This is important because nutrient deficiencies can play a role in stress, anxiety, and mood symptoms too.

For example, symptoms of a B vitamin deficiency can include nervousness, headaches, rapid heartbeat, difficulty concentrating, fatigue, and irritability... which are similar to symptoms of stress and anxiety. In fact, studies have found that low vitamin B6 and low iron levels contribute to panic attacks and anxiety in women. (30) Some experts also say vitamin B12 deficiency can cause almost any psychiatric symptom—from anxiety and panic to depression and hallucinations. (31)

Vitamin B9 (Folic Acid) deficiencies can also contribute (in a round-about way) because B9 metabolizes homocysteine and keeps those levels low. Why is that important? Because Homocysteine is inflammatory and neurotoxic. So, if it isn't broken down properly and builds up in the body, it can increase the risk of stroke, heart disease, free radical damage, and mitochondrial damage. It can also reduce energy production in the brain and lead to depression. (32) So Folic Acid is a crucial tool in keeping homocysteine levels down and mood up.

As already mentioned, though, not everyone can use Folic Acid, because up to 50% of the population has an MTHFR gene mutation, passed down from parents, which inhibits the use of this vitamin. (33) Some even say an MTHFR mutation is present in 98% of those with autism. (34)

Other factors can also interfere with how the body converts folic acid. For example, active thyroid hormones are needed for MTHFR function. That means having hypothyroidism can make the conversion difficult regardless of a gene mutation. Alcohol, candida, cow's milk, and medications (like metformin, oral contraceptives, lamotrigine, and antacids) can sometimes interfere with methylation too.

In addition, xFactor Plus also contains other vitamins and minerals that are needed to make and use other hormones. For example, it has 100% of the DV of Pantothenic acid (vitamin B5) which is needed to make both sex hormones and stress hormones, 150% of the DV of selenium which is needed to convert T4 into T3 and assist the adrenal glands, 500 mcg of boron which is needed for the body to use estrogen and testosterone, and 7000% of vitamin B12, which is needed for the adrenal system, nervous system, cardiovascular system, hormonal balance, enzyme production, and DNA synthesis.

In fact, xFactor Plus has methylcobalamin, which is the most absorbable form of vitamin B12. Because it is so absorbable, it can potentially stay in the body longer and at higher levels than cyanocobalamin, the other less absorbable form of vitamin B12. This can make it especially useful for people with Celiac disease and other digestive issues which we covered earlier in this book. Discuss this possibility with your doctor first.

Magnesium

When the body goes into "fight or flight" mode, it needs to be "stirred" for action, and so it flushes calming or sedative minerals like magnesium from the body and hangs on to stimulating ones. For this reason, the magnesium-containing Plexus Bio Cleanse™ could prove beneficial for those suffering from chronic stress. Though again, magnesium can interfere with some medications, so it is essential to talk to your doctor first.

What's more, when the stress response is ongoing digestion is put on hold, so minerals like potassium, sodium, and phosphorus can build up in the body, and can be re-absorbed by the kidneys. If you remember, minerals need to be balanced, so this can contribute to mineral imbalances. For more on this see phase 1.

Slim

As I mentioned before, visceral fat, or belly fat, not only acts as an endocrine organ with many cortisol receptors, it also converts inactive cortisol to active cortisol, creating a vicious cycle of stress and weight. From this, we see that to break the chronic stress response cycle, you have to get rid of visceral fat.

A tool that may help with this is Plexus Slim®. I have already discussed the many benefits of Slim® in previous phases, but it's worth reminding you of its effect on fat, especially visceral fat. Plexus Slim® contains an ingredient called Garcinia Cambogia which has been shown to significantly reduce visceral fat in a double-blind, randomized human study of men and women ages 20-65. (35)

Plexus Slim® also contains Alpha Lipoic Acid and Chlorogenic Acid, both of which have been shown to reduce visceral fat also. (36) (37)

Referernces:

(1) https://www.umms.org/ummc/patients-visitors/health-library/in-depth-patient-education-reports/articles/stress
(2) https://www.ncbi.nlm.nih.gov/pubmed/24153250
(3) https://www.ncbi.nlm.nih.gov/pmc/articles/PMC3942672/
(4) https://www.ncbi.nlm.nih.gov/pmc/articles/PMC4263906/
(5) http://www.apa.org/helpcenter/stress-body.aspx
(6) https://www.ncbi.nlm.nih.gov/pubmed/16353426
(7) https://www.sciencedaily.com/releases/2000/11/001120072314.htm
(8) http://journals.sagepub.com/doi/pdf/10.1177/2047487313492631
(9) https://www.ncbi.nlm.nih.gov/pubmed/18367704
(10) https://www.ncbi.nlm.nih.gov/pubmed/27573429.
(11) https://www.ncbi.nlm.nih.gov/pubmed/14618117
(12) https://www.ncbi.nlm.nih.gov/pmc/articles/PMC3181836/
(13) https://www.psychologytoday.com/us/blog/the-aftermath-trauma/201606/cortisol-and-ptsd-part-1
(14) https://www.barna.com/research/americans-feel-good-counseling/
(15) https://www.ncbi.nlm.nih.gov/pubmed/18787373
(16) https://www.ncbi.nlm.nih.gov/pmc/articles/PMC1332084/
(17) https://www.ncbi.nlm.nih.gov/pubmed/20129404
(18) https://www.ncbi.nlm.nih.gov/pmc/articles/PMC4203918/
(19) https://bemindful.co.uk/evidence-research/
(20) http://www.apa.org/monitor/2012/07-08/ce-corner.aspx
(21) https://www.psychologytoday.com/us/articles/200307/the-dangers-loneliness
(22) https://www.npr.org/sections/health-shots/2017/03/06/518362255/feeling-lonely-too-much-time-on-social-media-may-be-why
(23) https://www.sciencedirect.com/science/article/pii/S2352289516300509
(24) https://www.ncbi.nlm.nih.gov/pmc/articles/PMC5102282/
(25) https://www.ncbi.nlm.nih.gov/pmc/articles/PMC4410136/
(26) https://www.sciencedirect.com/science/article/pii/S0166223616301138
(27) https://www.hindawi.com/journals/ijmicro/2016/8469018/
(28) https://www.ncbi.nlm.nih.gov/pubmed/26620542

(29) https://www.ucc.ie/en/media/academic/psychiatry/Allen_NeuroIreland_2015_Bif Longum.pdf
(30) https://www.ncbi.nlm.nih.gov/pubmed/23603926
(31) https://www.psychologytoday.com/us/blog/health-matters/201202/vitamin-b12
(32) https://www.ncbi.nlm.nih.gov/pubmed/17541043
(33) https://www.dietvsdisease.org/mthfr-mutation-symptoms-and-diet/
(34) https://www.drrodneyrussell.com/what-is-mthfr/
(35) https://www.ncbi.nlm.nih.gov/pmc/articles/PMC4053034/
(36) https://www.ncbi.nlm.nih.gov/pubmed/27276401
(37) https://www.ncbi.nlm.nih.gov/pubmed/16545124

Phase 8:

Rebuilding the Exterior

Materials: Filtered Water, Carrots, Sweet Potatoes, Nuts, Seeds, Seafood, Eggs, and Leafy Greens

Tools: xFactor Plus™, Slim®, Plexus Body Cream, and Joyōme®

225

Chapter 14: The Curb Appeal of Youthful Skin

The exterior of a house is often referred to as its "curb appeal." It's how the house looks on the outside—and usually involves things like siding or shingles, the paint, etc. The exterior of the temple of the body is similar. It includes how the body looks—usually referring to skincare, and things like wrinkles, sunspots, blemishes, etc.

When it comes to *improving* skin, it's like trying to improve the exterior of a house. To some, it might seem as though the exterior is just "for show." But actually, the exterior of a house is very important to the overall state of the home. Without quality siding (or solid stone, brick, or wood) the underlying boards, insulation, wiring, etc. are vulnerable to damage. The exterior is a protective barrier. It also helps regulate the temperature inside the home, because a faulty exterior can let in cold or hot air.

Likewise, your skin (the body's largest organ) has a some "pretty" important jobs to do. It helps regulate internal body temperature, and it protects you from harmful things like toxins and germs. Without skin, you'd be an open gate to infection and illness.

But your skin is still so much more than even that. It's capable of so many different jobs. For example, unlike siding or brick, your skin is a two-way street, so to speak. Skin keeps harmful things from entering the body, yes, but it also pulls out harmful things too. Your skin is an amazing detoxification organ that expels detrimental substances through your pores, via sweat. Think of it as a porous sponge... it can soak water up and squeeze water out.

Your skin also has multiple layers (3 main ones, to be exact) which are similar to the way a house has three exterior layers: boards, shingles, and paint. Each layer serves a purpose and function.

What's even more amazing is that your skin has its own ecosystem living on it. It's called the skin microbiome. It's similar to the gut microbiome in that it is a collection of numerous good and bad bacteria conducting many important "temple" jobs. Think of it as if your house had a layer of bugs (good ones and bad ones) living on the siding. The bad ones try to damage the home like carpenter ants, but the good ones act like pest control, devouring the bad ones. Not enough good ones enable the bad ones to run rampant on the house.

As you can see the exterior of your temple is so much more than just curb appeal. (Your skin is so much more than beauty.) Therefore, to address curb appeal, we really have to address the exterior on all its levels.

You can slap up a new coat of paint on your house but if your boards underneath are moldy or warped is that *really* fixing anything? Such is the case with the skin. True and lasting beauty often comes from within.

The Skin-Gut Connection

One of the first and most important things to consider when trying to maintain healthy skin is to maintain a healthy gut. This is perhaps one of the most overlooked aspects of any beauty regimen. But in my opinion, it is probably the most crucial. It boils down to two factors. One, nutrient absorption and two, gut dysbiosis.

Let's start with nutrients. If you aren't getting (or absorbing) the nutrients that your skin needs, the skin will start to show it. Here are my top five most important nutrients for maintaining healthy skin:

#1 Vitamin A:

There are two forms of vitamin A (retinoids, or retinol, and carotenoids). Retinol is the *usable* or "bioavailable" form of vitamin A, and it's found mostly in animal foods. Carotenoids are precursors, meaning the body will convert them to retinol vitamin A, and they are mostly in plant foods like carrots and sweet potatoes. Both forms of vitamin A are important for different reasons. Retinol (which is a fat-soluble vitamin) helps skin cell production and promotes fibroblast cells—which help keep skin firm. It also stimulates collagen production, which can reduce wrinkles.

Carotenoids are water-soluble and are antioxidants that can protect cells from UV rays, prevent cell damage and premature aging. And, as I said, they can be converted into retinol... that is if you are healthy. If you have gut/digestive issues, your body might not do this efficiently. Also, if you do not eat animal foods, this could increase the likelihood of retinol deficiency, as can alcoholism and sugar addiction because vitamin A is stored in the liver which often becomes damaged after years of heavy drinking and high sugar.

#2 Vitamin E:

Vitamin E is also a fat-soluble vitamin and one of the most powerful antioxidants around. It's found in foods such as nuts, seeds, and leafy greens. It powerfully combats free radicals and the cell/skin damage that can occur from them. In fact, studies have shown that vitamin E reduces eczema and psoriasis symptoms, and also reduces scars and speeds wound healing. It also can prevent sunburn, moisturize dry skin, and prevent/reduce wrinkles.

#3 Selenium:

Selenium has antioxidant properties too and works in conjunction with vitamin E (even increasing the effectiveness of vitamin E). Like vitamin E, selenium works against free radicals, protecting cells from damage, before wrinkles show up. It actually helps form a coating around cells to protect them and preserves the skin's elasticity. Selenium is found in foods such as eggs, brazil nuts, sunflower seeds, and seafood.

#4 Zinc:

Zinc is a trace mineral with anti-inflammatory and antioxidant properties too. It's needed by every cell in the body—especially the skin—because it is used for cell production and turnover. It is most abundant in the outer layer of the skin, and it also helps make collagen. Zinc is found most heavily in oysters, red meat, and poultry, but dairy, beans, and nuts also have moderate amounts.

#5 Omega 3s:

As I've mentioned before, omega 3 fatty acids are enormously important in the health of the cell, because the outside layer of a cell membrane is made up mostly of Omega 3s. And the cell membrane is what holds moisture in the cell. Put simply, if the cell membrane is not strong or it is damaged, it won't hold water. If it doesn't hold water, your skin won't be well hydrated, which means it won't be smooth and soft. (This is why hydration is another key to healthy skin. Rule of thumb: we should be drinking half our body weight in ounces of water each day.)

Omega 3s are also anti-inflammatory—and inflammation is super hard on your skin. The purpose of inflammation is your body's way of dealing with a foreign invader or injury. It initiates inflammation in an attempt to destroy damaged or infected cells so that new, healthy cells can begin to form.

The problem is when the body suffers chronic inflammation from things like stress, allergies, etc. the body is continually breaking down cells. After a while, it starts breaking down collagen fibers too—which contributes greatly to wrinkles and other signs of aging.

So the bottom line is this: your outside glow often starts INSIDE, with your nutrients!! If your digestion is compromised or you think you might not be getting enough from your diet, you may want to consider supplementing with a quality multi-vitamin like xFactor Plus™ and an omega supplement.

The Skin Microbiome

The second "gut factor" that might hinder a healthy "glow" is gut dysbiosis. I've already talked extensively about the gut microbiome (the trillions of microbes that live in the digestive tract) and all the important jobs these bacteria do in the body. But what is important to remember is that "dysbiosis" (having more bad guys than good guys) can dramatically impact your skin too. There is a direct correlation between an unhealthy gut and skin issues such as eczema, rosacea, psoriasis, and acne.

Take, for example, leaky gut. If the intestinal lining becomes damaged, food particles and toxins can slip out into the bloodstream, where they don't belong, which can cause an immune reaction. The immune system might think misplaced food is a foreign substance and send out antibodies to get rid of it. The antibodies could then make histamine, which irritates the skin. This is why it's not uncommon for food allergies and sensitivities to be the underlying root cause of many skin irritations.

What's more, your skin has its own microbiome. There are more than 1 trillion tiny little microbes (bacteria, fungi, yeasts, and viruses) living on the surface of your skin and in deeper layers. These good guys and bad guys come from more than 1,000 different species, and they help keep your skin healthy.

Ideally, these microbes will encourage a slightly acidic skin pH, which helps to prevent infections and retain moisture, keeping skin soft and smooth. These microbes can work with the immune system to control skin inflammation, and they even help heal sun damage and begin wound healing.

As we all know, there comes a point in life when our skin begins to show signs of aging. Like the exterior of a house, the exterior of your temple can also suffer natural "wear and tear" with age and exposure to the elements. Not only does our skin get thinner with age, but environmental, lifestyle, and chemical factors contribute, too. These can affect multiple layers of the skin in multiple ways.

The Many Layers

The first layer of the skin (even though it isn't technically a "layer") is the skin microbiome, the microbial army that protects you from illness and infection. This is your skin's first line of defense, so to speak, but it is not restricted to just the outside layer. Microbes are actually found in all layers of the skin, even the deep fat layers. And each species has an important job to do to keep you healthy and looking your best. So, if the skin microbiome is disrupted—if the balance between good and bad microbes is upset—bacterial overgrowths, yeast infections, and viral infections can occur. These can result in rashes and discoloration.

If the skin microbiome is disrupted, the pH of the skin could change too. I've talked about pH before, but what's important to remember in terms of skincare is that pH refers to the amount of hydrogen in water… and our skin is made up of mostly water, so this is important. If your skin pH becomes too alkaline, it can lead to dryness, flaking, irritation, and yes, more wrinkles.

What are some things that can harm the skin microbiome? Ironically, antimicrobial products! Hand sanitizer, which is designed to kill microbes, causes skin dysbiosis! Soaps (hand soap and bar soap) are by their very nature alkalizing (and remember your skin should be acidic). A healthy skin pH should be somewhere around five (under seven is acidic, over seven alkaline). However, most bar soaps have a pH of about 10! That's very alkaline.

Why is this a problem? Because many harmful bacteria thrive in alkaline environments, but good bacteria thrive in acidic environments. Therefore, that bar soap your slathering on your face every day could be making it very difficult to maintain the proper pH your microbes need to retain moisture, fight infection, and support the immune system.

The First Real Layer

The top, outermost layer of the skin is an oily layer where fats and waxes reside. It is a protective barrier. If this becomes damaged, the skin will be less able to hold moisture in, and it will also become less "elastic." In other words, when you smile, laugh, or frown (and your skin creases and folds) it will have a harder time "bouncing back" from those expressions, and lines and wrinkles can form where those facial expressions occurred.

What can damage this outer layer of the skin? Sun exposure is among the most common, which can result in not just wrinkles, but also sun spots and discoloration. Other things that can be detrimental to the outer layer: harsh chemicals found in beauty products, lotions, and cleansers, as well as overly hot water (it's important to wash with warm or lukewarm water, not hot water).

Damage Beneath the Surface

The most common factor that affects the deeper layer of skin is UV light. Extended sun exposure (or tanning beds) not only affects the outer layer of the skin, but it can also weaken the collagen and connective tissue beneath the skin's surface which gives skin its structure. This can make skin weaker, structurally, and therefore cause it to sag and develop those deep wrinkles and folds that are especially hard to get rid of.

Smoking can also damage the deeper layers of skin. Smoking not only releases toxins into the body which damage skin cells, but it also makes it harder to get oxygen to these cells (which your skin needs to heal, repair, and regenerate new and healthy cells).

Perhaps at this point, you might be thinking you need to beef up your supply of beauty products to protect yourself from all this potential skin weakening and damage. While that is probably the case, yes, please don't just head out to the local drugstore or department store and buy one of the most expensive products they offer in the hopes it will do the trick. Often these "miracle products" only make skin worse. Allow me to explain.

Typical beauty products contain a lot of chemicals that not only irritate and dry out the skin but also can contribute to more serious issues.

The average woman puts anywhere from 150 to 515 synthetic chemicals on her body every single day without even knowing it. From lotions, hair care, makeup, fragrance, you name it. The skin is the largest organ of the body, and because it is porous, it absorbs whatever is put on it. In fact, almost 70% of what we put onto our skin is absorbed into our bodies! It goes directly into the bloodstream in most cases.

Why is this a problem? Because many of the chemicals in beauty products are toxic. The European Union has banned over 1,300 chemicals found in cosmetics, but the FDA has only banned eight and restricted three. Therefore, many chemicals are still being used here in America in common, everyday products.

Below is a list of the most common (and detrimental) chemicals found in many cleansers, lotions, makeup, and other beauty products.

- Sodium lauryl sulfate is a lung irritant that can disrupt your skin's oil balance
- Aminophenol, Phenylenediamine, and Diaminobenzene come from coal tar, which is a known carcinogen. Enough said.
- Benzoyl peroxide is antimicrobial, disrupting the skin microbiome
- BHA is a carcinogen, hormone disruptor, and affects the pigment of the skin
- Triclosan and triclocarban disrupts the skin microbiome and hormone balance
- Polyethylene (also called PEGs) are carcinogens and skin irritants used as "penetration enhancers," meaning they increase the skin's absorption (which is not good if there are other harmful ingredients too)
- The term "fragrance" or "parfum" are often umbrella terms for hormone-disrupting chemicals, many of which are carcinogens.
- Parabens (anything that ends in "araben") mimic estrogen and can, therefore, disrupt hormone balance. In fact, a recent study found parabens in 99% of breast cancer tumors studied. (1)
- Synthetic colors are often derived from petroleum or coal tar sources, which are known carcinogens
- Phthalates are hormone disruptors and have been linked to breast cancer
- Formaldehyde-releasing preservatives (FRP's) disrupt the microbiome and are allergens and carcinogens
- DEA (diethanolamine) disrupts the pH of the skin microbiome
- Propylene glycol is an alcohol and skin irritant associated with dermatitis and hives
- Toluene is a petroleum and coal tar derivative that is so strong it can dissolve paint
- Siloxanes are endocrine disruptors that also affect brain neurotransmitters. These can bioaccumulate too, meaning they are not easily expelled from the body and tend to build up in tissue

Joyōme®

I know the above list can seem disheartening, but there *is* a way to moisturize your skin without a ton of chemicals while feeding the skin microbiome at the same time. My absolute favorite tools for this kind of project are the Plexus Joyōme® skincare products. Plexus Joyōme® is not a complicated regimen, like some other products. It involves just two easy steps—moisturize in the morning with the day serum and moisturize again at night with the overnight repair serum.

What makes Joyōme® really unique, though, is its absorption abilities. Sometimes, beauty products don't thoroughly soak in and are left resting on the skin's surface. But Joyōme® contains a patented HydraLipid Delivery System that increases absorption. Plant-derived fats act as ingredient carriers, transporting them down through the skin's tough outer layer... whereas other products use *synthetic* delivery ingredients that are not as safe or gentle.

What's more, when making Joyōme®, Plexus left out every ingredient on the EU's banned list, as well as more than 1,300 other questionable ingredients too, including harmful fragrances. Instead, Plexus uses botanically-based, essential oils such as damask rose oil from Bulgaria, and essential oils of vanilla, ylang-ylang, lavender, and marjoram that have an uplifting scent and help enhance the beauty of the skin.

In other words, Joyōme® is uncommonly clean.

The Illuminating Day Serum

The Joyōme® Illuminating Day Serum contains six key ingredients to help reverse the visible signs of aging, as well as a light-reflecting pigment to give skin a glowing, radiant look.

1. Argireline Peptide – Reduces the appearance of wrinkles associated with repetitive facial expressions, especially in the forehead and around the eyes
2. Hyaluronic Acid (HA) – Improves the appearance of sagging, drooping skin by helping it to look plump and tight
3. Red Clover – Minimizes the appearance of pores by reducing oil accumulation and pore debris
4. Niacinamide – Helps with skin brightening
5. Eyeseryl Peptide – Reduces the appearance of puffiness and dark circles under the eyes
6. Ceramides – Help to lock in moisture and reduce the appearance of wrinkles

Intensive Overnight Repair

The Joyōme® Intensive Overnight Repair serum contains five key ingredients to help you wake up to skin that looks firmer, lushly moisturized, and beautifully smooth.

1. Retinoid Ester* – Reduces the appearance of deep lines and wrinkles, visible age spots, and renews the appearance of skin plumpness, elasticity, and hydration
2. Matrixyl Peptide – Helps to fill and smooth the skin
3. Azelaic Acid – Visibly fades the appearance of redness, age spots and improves the look of skin texture to reveal luminous, radiant skin
4. Lactic Acid – Helps exfoliate dead surface cells leading to more radiant, smooth, glowing skin
5. Bakuchiol – Conditions the skin and helps to improve skin clarity

* Retinoid Ester is different than traditional retinol. First, a retinoid ester (versus retinol) does not need to undergo biochemical changes to become active on the skin. Second, a retinoid ester is ten times more stable than retinol, so it has a longer potency (compared to traditional retinol, which breaks down quickly with light, heat, and time). Third, retinoid ester has a unique delivery system (dimethyl isosorbide), that allows it to reach the areas of the skin where it's needed most.

The Skin Microbiome

Both Joyōme® products contain a patent-pending Microbiome Balancing Complex that uses the skin's own good microbes as well as polyphenols and prebiotics to bring the skin microbiome into balance. In fact, this complex has been scientifically shown to increase the beneficial microbe *S. epidermidis* and crowd out the unwanted microbe *S. aureus*.

S. epidermidis is a good skin microbe that works to replenish the skin barrier, allowing the skin to retain moisture while defending it from damaging environmental factors. S. aureus, on the other hand, weakens the skin barrier, making it susceptible to dryness and dullness. Also, the Beta-glucan contained in the complex hinders this unwanted microbe from adhering to the skin, further defending the skin from damage.

The Data is In!

An eight-week clinical study was conducted by an outside research center that followed thirty-two women, ages 35 to 65 and of varying ethnicities and skin types, to see how Joyōme® delivered results. At the end of eight weeks, subjects underwent a series of clinical measurements using computerized evaluation tools, including a sophisticated 3-D facial mapping camera. Joyōme® improved the appearance of all visible signs of aging. Below are the actual results. There were no adverse events or irritation observed on any subject during the study

- A total of 97%, 88% and 100% of the subjects showed improvement in the appearance of global facial fine lines/wrinkles 1, 4 and 8 weeks of product use, respectively
- A total of 41%, 53% and 91% of the subjects showed improvement in under-eye puffiness following 1, 4 and 8 weeks of product use, respectively
- A total of 88%, 66% and 91% of the subjects showed improvement in skin elasticity after 1, 4, and 8 weeks of use, respectively.
- A total of 100% of the subjects showed improvement in hydration skin immediately following a single-use and after 1, 4 and 8 weeks of use
- A total of 97%, 88%, and 100% of the subjects showed improvement in facial pore size 1, 4, and 8 weeks of product use, respectively.

Plexus® Body Cream

When it comes to full-body hydration, I also use the very-clean Plexus® Body Cream. The ingredients that I love most are:

- The Oil Blend: Plexus® Body Cream contains a blend of five different oils—sweet almond oil, grape seed oil, evening primrose oil, lavender oil, and Rosaceae oil—to help.
- Spirulina Algae: This blue-green algae purifies the skin, fights free radicals, and encourages faster cell turnover to enable skin healing. It is also a good source of chlorophyll, as I mentioned before, which can help the skin retain its moisture.
- Activated Charcoal: This a charcoal powder that has been heated at high temperatures to "activate" it. This means it has a negative electrical charge that attracts things like toxins which are positively charged, thus making it beneficial in cleansing the skin and body.
- Aloe Vera Gel: The stems of the aloe vera plant store water, which creates a gel in its leaves. This gel contains approximately 75 different ingredients, such as antioxidants, vitamins, minerals, and amino acids. Many of these are anti-viral and anti-fungal, and they can also help cells regenerate, making it very beneficial in skincare.

References

(1) https://articles.mercola.com/sites/articles/archive/2012/04/02/toxic-parabens-on-breast-cancer-patients.aspx

Chapter 15: The Beginning

Disclaimer: These statements have not been evaluated by the Food and Drug Administration. None of the information in this book is intended to diagnose, treat, cure, or prevent any disease. All information contained in this chapter and this book are for educational purposes only and are not intended to replace the advice of a medical doctor. Stacy Malesiewski is not a doctor and does not give medical advice, prescribe medication, or diagnose illness. Stacy is a certified health coach, journalist, and an independent Plexus ambassador. These are her personal beliefs and are not the beliefs of Plexus Worldwide, Gray Matter Media, Inc., or any other named professionals in this book. If you have a medical condition or health concern, it is advised that you see your physician immediately. It is also recommended that you consult your doctor before implementing any new health strategy or taking any new supplements. Results may vary

The last time my husband and I moved, we did an immense amount of work on our home before calling the realtor. I don't think there was an area in our house (inside or outside) that didn't experience some sort of renovation. We worked our tails off and spent a lot of money. But, in the end, we felt good about the effort we put into it. We felt accomplished, proud, excited, and ready.

The house looked gorgeous. So gorgeous, that we wondered why we didn't do it sooner. The photos in our online listing were almost unrecognizable. And our first open house attracted more than 13 families!

At that point, we decided to put new "family rules" in place. First rule: no more carpet-ruining, sofa-staining "slime" for our kids. (If you don't know what slime is, it's the devil's toy. A gooey, messy version of silly putty that destroys almost anything it touches.)

Second rule: Scooters are hereby for <u>outdoor</u> use only. (I know, this seems obvious. But our downstairs was shaped like a circular racetrack. It's quite tempting.) Third rule: Markers are to be used at the craft table only—and never, EVER on walls, doors, or floors. (Again, this probably seems like a no-brainer, but my six-year-old is a magician and graffiti master.)

Anyway, there were many, other, similar rules put in place, but they were all to ensure the same result: that our house stayed in the condition we worked so hard to get it to.

Are you following me, here? Do you see where I am going with this?

You've arrived at the end of this book. For most of you, though, this probably isn't the <u>*end*</u> of your personal renovation. You're probably not finished rebuilding your temple yet. In fact, you could just be getting started. But at some point, you might start accomplishing various health goals. Like my husband and I after our home renovations, you might start feeling accomplished and proud of the work you've put into this. You might start feeling excited about what else is in store. You might even start loving your new online photos!

If this happens, it's important to stop and think back on the things that may have contributed to the unhealthy state you were in when you first decided to rebuild. Consider the things that had the most damaging effect on your health – a soda addiction, processed food, too much sugar, smoking, alcohol, not enough sleep, a sedentary lifestyle, unmanaged stress, or a combination of various things.

Identify the lifestyle factors that may have hurt your health and then set up temple rules so you can avoid those in the future. Also, come up with a backup plan for when the temptation comes.

For example, rule number one in our new, post-reno home was "no slime for our kids." Slime had done so much damage that we just banned it altogether. The problem is, slime is (or was) the latest rage amongst kids everywhere. It was given as birthday favors and presents; they made it with their friends in art class; other kids would come to sleepovers with jars of it packed in their overnight bag. There are even whole YouTube channels devoted to the messy gunk! Slime, unfortunately, was inescapable.

So, we had to reevaluate rule number one. We had to accept the fact that we couldn't avoid it forever. We decided that while we weren't going to actively purchase slime for our kids, we would allow it when it was given to them as a gift, or on special occasions. However, the kids would have to play with it in their metal playhouse, outside in the yard. Slime was not to be played with in our home or even *stored* in our home.

The same might be true for 'post-reno you.' You might have identified several damaging lifestyle habits throughout this rebuilding process—you might have even successfully overcome them. But, now it is time to set up rules for yourself so that you don't revert back to those old, damaging habits and undo all your hard work.

Perhaps you quit your nightly bowl of ice cream cold turkey and haven't had a lick of ice cream in a month. Kudos to you! I'm so proud of you! But, friend, chances are ice cream (like slime) will show it's ugly (yet tempting) face at some point. You probably won't be able to avoid it forever. So how will you handle that? What's your game plan?

Perhaps (like our slime rule) you'll need to make a rule that ice cream doesn't get stored in the house (it's too tempting). But maybe it can be enjoyed on special occasions _outside_ of the house—like, say, at an event or a friend's birthday—maybe even with some Plexus Block or a Plexus Slim pink drink beforehand.

The point is: it's important to be real with yourself. You're human. You'll be tempted. And you'll want to cave. Caving is OK, though—occasionally. (Unless we are talking about addiction, which is an entirely different story.) Caving "here and there," though, that is called living. Balanced living. Caving for a *week* or *month* straight, on the other hand, is called a habit. And it's the *habits* (the *bad* habits) that we want to avoid, because they are what often cause the most damage.

So, now that you've arrived at the end of this book—now that you've identified those lifestyle factors that were not good for you, and have educated yourself on *how* to rebuild your temple—begin to develop a game plan for how you will resist the temptations to go back to those old unhealthy ways. If you need help with this, I offer suggestions in the *Rebuilding Your Temple workbook*.

And please don't blow this off. This is a crucial part of *maintaining* your health. This is what differentiates yo-yo diets from complete lifestyle changes. This is often what separates people who constantly fluctuate back and forth (between healthy and unhealthy) from the people who successfully transform their lives. It's the ability to be real with yourself, to *enjoy* living, to practice balance, and to be disciplined.

The Movement

While my husband and I were making renovations to our home, it often happened that friends, family, or neighbors would inquire about the work we were doing: *Hey, your front door looks great, how did you refinish it? I love the new perennials out front, what are they called? That new barn wood accent wall is so cute, how did you do it?*

The people in our life were taking notice of the work we were doing and asking questions. Unknowingly, we were encouraging others to put in a little elbow grease too, and they started making their own renovations. After a while, it seemed like our whole community was undergoing a renovation of some sort.

This also happens (a lot) when people start rebuilding their temples. So be prepared. Coworkers might see you eating salads or drinking a pink drink. Friends might start to notice that you look thinner. Family might take note of your new mood and energy level. If this happens, they might start asking questions about what you're doing and how you're rebuilding. At that point, you have two options.

One: you could play coy, shrug it off, and pretend it's nothing. If you're not a talker, or not comfortable discussing your personal life with others, you might want to just keep quiet.

Two: you could step out of your comfort zone and tell them a little bit about *Rebuilding Your Temple* and what you've been doing. Sure, it might seem easier to say nothing. But if your friend, coworker, family member, or neighbor is struggling, you might be able to encourage them to rebuild with their doctor too. They then might encourage their family and friends also, who might encourage their family and friends, and so forth and so on.

In this way, you might become part of a Rebuilding *movement*! Think about that for a minute. Please. Remember the statistics I gave you at the beginning of this book.

Almost 40% of U.S. adults are now classified as obese. (1) More than 90 million Americans have been diagnosed with Cardiovascular Disease. (2) Nearly 40% of men and women will be diagnosed with cancer at some point during their lifetimes. (3) Approximately 50 million Americans (20% of the population, or one in five people) suffer from one or more of the now 80 classified autoimmune diseases. (4) More than 100 million U.S. adults are now living with diabetes or prediabetes. (5) And nearly 70% of Americans are taking at least one prescription drug (and more than half of the population is taking two). (6)

In addition to the devastating effects these issues have on individuals and families, they also have a massive effect on our country as a whole. U.S. health care spending grew 3.9 percent in 2017, reaching $3.5 trillion or $10,739 per person. (7) In fact, the United States spends more on health care than the rest of the world combined. (8) Yet, somehow, we are not healthier.

In one study, researchers examined international data comparing the U.S. with ten other high-income countries. Life expectancy was the lowest in the U.S., and we spent nearly twice as much on drugs, per person, as the other countries in the study. (9)

You might be frustrated by these statistics; you might even feel hopeless in the face of them. The increasing mortality rates and the declining health of our country might seem like a big political issue that is far beyond your control. You might think, *'What can little ol' me do to impact the scope of this giant problem?'*

I get it. You aren't a politician or a doctor. You don't serve on a medical board or work for the FDA. So you wonder what you can do to help the health of our nation. But, friend, you can do *your* part. You can educate yourself on what your body needs. Then you can make diet and lifestyle changes to positively affect your health—and you can encourage others to do the same.

This is especially important if you are a parent! Start, first and foremost, by encouraging those in your own home. Let's face it: parents determine the food children eat. They purchase it, cook it, pack it in lunches, and even choose which restaurants the family will eat at. Understand that parents have a dual responsibility to their own personal health as well as that of the next generation—which, right now, is gravely threatened.

Experts contend that, for the first time in history, the next generation may not live longer than their parents, due to obesity-related diseases that are largely *preventable*. (10) (11) This should sound like a battle cry for parents everywhere. (For information on how to help your children get healthy, watch for the *Rebuilding Little Temples* series and the *Rebuilding Your Temple Homeschool Edition* textbook and workbook coming soon.)

Consider this your summoning, your call, your invitation to fight for the health of your family and your country. In my opinion, friends, we won't win this battle in the political arena or the board room, but rather, in the kitchen and in the grocery store aisles—in a grassroots effort to eat and live healthier.

Let's face it: food manufacturers are only going to produce what the majority of consumers buy. So, when more people buy healthy options, the more healthy options they will produce. The same is true when it comes to healthier options for beauty products, household cleaners, and so on. The consumer drives the market.

Friend, that means *you*.

<u>You</u> are in the driver's seat here. You have a responsibility and a role to play when it comes to the health of our nation and our world. And by completing this book, you've already taken the first step—education.

Where will you go from here, though? Will you soon close up this book, continue rebuilding for another month, and then go back to your old ways as soon as you fit into those size eight jeans? Will you keep this information to yourself and never speak of it to anyone?

 Or… will you share this information with your coworkers, neighbors, friends, and family? Will you start a *Rebuilding Your Temple* small group study and encourage others to educate themselves too? Will you enforce healthier eating habits in your house and teach your kids what their bodies need? Will you continue to make healthy diet and lifestyle choices in your own life, serving as a role model and leader in your home and your community?

This might be the end of the book, but my friend, this is just the beginning of the movement.

Education is meant to be shared and passed on…like a small flame spreading from person to person. Sure, the earlier statistics might seem gloomy and dark. But the torch is in your hands now. What will you do with it? Don't let it burn out in a month or two. Begin to set other hearts on fire now.

This is how we will rebuild the health of our world—one temple at a time.

References:

(1) https://www.cdc.gov/obesity/data/adult.html
(2) http://www.acc.org/latest-in-cardiology/ten-points-to-remember/2017/02/09/14/58/heart-disease-and-stroke-statistics-2017
(3) https://www.cancer.gov/about-cancer/understanding/statistics
(4) https://www.aarda.org/knowledge-base/many-americans-autoimmune-disease/
(5) https://www.cdc.gov/media/releases/2017/p0718-diabetes-report.html
(6) https://newsnetwork.mayoclinic.org/discussion/nearly-7-in-10-americans-take-prescription-drugs-mayo-clinic-olmsted-medical-center-find/
(7) https://www.cms.gov/research-statistics-data-and-systems/statistics-trends-and-reports/nationalhealthexpenddata/nationalhealthaccountshistorical.html
(8) http://www.hhpronline.org/articles/2018/10/8/increasing-mortality-and-declining-health-status-in-the-usa-where-is-public-health
(9) https://www.reuters.com/article/us-health-spending/u-s-health-spending-twice-other-countries-with-worse-results-idUSKCN1GP2YN
(10) https://medicalxpress.com/news/2011-01-obesity-children-life-short.html
(11) https://www.prb.org/willrisingchildhoodobesitydecreaseuslifeexpectancy/

INDEX

Triplex Dosing Schedule

Below is a sample of a Triplex dosing schedule that works for *some* people. Ask your doctor if this schedule is right for you, or if it needs to be adjusted (especially if you are taking any medications). Do not follow this protocol unless you have first consulted a licensed medical professional who has told you it is OK to do so.

Bio Cleanse dosage may vary. Bio Cleanse should not be increased once a daily, soft bowel movement is achieved. DO NOT ADD PROBIO5 to regimen until regularity is achieved. Repeat day 30 for 30 more days, if your doctor allows.

Disclaimer: These statements have not been evaluated by the Food and Drug Administration. None of the information in this book is intended to diagnose, treat, cure, or prevent any disease. All information contained in this chapter and this book are for educational purposes only and are not intended to replace the advice of a medical doctor. Stacy Malesiewski is not a doctor and does not give medical advice, prescribe medication, or diagnose illness. Stacy is a certified health coach, journalist, and an independent Plexus ambassador. These are her personal beliefs and are not the beliefs of Plexus Worldwide, Gray Matter Media, Inc., or any other named professionals in this book. If you have a medical condition or health concern, it is advised that you see your physician immediately. It is also recommended that you consult your doctor before implementing any new health strategy or taking any new supplements. Results may vary

DAY	A.M. BEFORE BREAKFAST	P.M. BEFORE DINNER OR BEDTIME
1	1 Slim	
2	1 Slim	
3	1 Slim	
4	1 Slim	
5	1 Slim	1 Bio Cleanse
6	1 Slim	1 Bio Cleanse
7	1 Slim and 1 ProBio 5	1 Bio Cleanse
8	1 Slim and 1 ProBio 5	1 Bio Cleanse
9	1 Slim and 1 ProBio 5	2 Bio Cleanse
10	1 Slim and 1 ProBio 5	2 Bio Cleanse
11	1 Slim and 2 ProBio 5	2 Bio Cleanse
12	1 Slim and 2 ProBio 5	2 Bio Cleanse
13	1 Slim and 2 ProBio 5	2 Bio Cleanse
14	1 Slim and 2 ProBio 5	3 Bio Cleanse
15	1 Slim and 3 ProBio 5	3 Bio Cleanse
16	1 Slim and 3 ProBio 5	3 Bio Cleanse
17	1 Slim and 3 ProBio 5	4 Bio Cleanse
18	1 Slim and 3 ProBio 5	4 Bio Cleanse

19	1 Slim and 3 ProBio 5	4 Bio Cleanse
20	1 Slim and 3 ProBio 5	4 Bio Cleanse
21	1 Slim and 3 ProBio 5	5 Bio Cleanse
22	1 Slim and 3 ProBio 5	5 Bio Cleanse
23	1 Slim and 4 ProBio 5	5 Bio Cleanse
24	1 Slim and 4 ProBio 5	5 Bio Cleanse
25	1 Slim and 4 ProBio 5	2 Bio Cleanse
26	1 Slim and 4 ProBio 5	2 Bio Cleanse
27	1 Slim and 4 ProBio 5	2 Bio Cleanse
28	1 Slim and 4 ProBio 5	2 Bio Cleanse
28	1 Slim and 4 ProBio 5	2 Bio Cleanse
30	1 Slim and 4 ProBio 5	2 Bio Cleanse

Triplex Autoimmune Dosing Schedule

Below is a sample of a Triplex dosing schedule that works for *some* people with Autoimmune issues. Ask your doctor if this schedule is right for you, or if it needs to be adjusted. Do not follow this protocol unless you have first consulted a licensed medical professional who has told you it is OK to do so.

Bio Cleanse dosage may vary. Bio Cleanse should not be increased once a daily, soft bowel movement is achieved. DO NOT ADD PROBIO5 to regimen until regularity is achieved. Repeat day 30 for 30 more days, if your doctor allows.

Disclaimer: These statements have not been evaluated by the Food and Drug Administration. None of the information in this book is intended to diagnose, treat, cure, or prevent any disease. All information contained in this chapter and this book are for educational purposes only and are not intended to replace the advice of a medical doctor. Stacy Malesiewski is not a doctor and does not give medical advice, prescribe medication, or diagnose illness. Stacy is a certified health coach, journalist, and an independent Plexus ambassador. These are her personal beliefs and are not the beliefs of Plexus Worldwide, Gray Matter Media, Inc., or any other named professionals in this book. If you have a medical condition or health concern, it is advised that you see your physician immediately. It is also recommended that you consult your doctor before implementing any new health strategy or taking any new supplements. Results may vary

DAY	A.M. BEFORE BREAKFAST	P.M. BEFORE DINNER	P.M BEFORE BEDTIME
1	1 Bio Cleanse		
2	1 Bio Cleanse		
3	1 Bio Cleanse		
4	1 Bio Cleanse	1 Bio Cleanse	
5	1 Bio Cleanse	1 Bio Cleanse	
6	1 Bio Cleanse	1 Bio Cleanse	
7	1 Bio Cleanse	1 Bio Cleanse	
8	½ Slim and 1 Bio Cleanse	1 Bio Cleanse	
9	½ Slim and 1 Bio Cleanse	1 Bio Cleanse	
10	½ Slim and 1 Bio Cleanse	1 Bio Cleanse	
11	½ Slim and 1 Bio Cleanse	1 Bio Cleanse	
12	1 Slim and 1 Bio Cleanse	1 Bio Cleanse	

DAY	A.M. BEFORE BREAKFAST	P.M. BEFORE DINNER	P.M BEFORE BEDTIME
13	1 Slim and 1 Bio Cleanse	1 Bio Cleanse	
14	1 Slim and 1 Bio Cleanse	1 Bio Cleanse	
15	1 Slim and 1 Bio Cleanse	1 Bio Cleanse	
16	1 Slim and 2 Bio Cleanse	1 Bio Cleanse	
17	1 Slim and 2 Bio Cleanse	1 Bio Cleanse	
18	1 Slim and 2 Bio Cleanse	1 Bio Cleanse	
19	1 Slim and 2 Bio Cleanse	1 Bio Cleanse	
20	1 Slim and 2 Bio Cleanse	2 Bio Cleanse	
21	1 Slim and 2 Bio Cleanse	2 Bio Cleanse	
22	1 Slim and 2 Bio Cleanse	2 Bio Cleanse	
23	1 Slim and 2 Bio Cleanse	2 Bio Cleanse	
24	1 Slim and 2 Bio Cleanse	2 Bio Cleanse	1 ProBio5
25	1 Slim and 2 Bio Cleanse	2 Bio Cleanse	1 ProBio5
26	1 Slim and 2 Bio Cleanse	2 Bio Cleanse	1 ProBio5
27	1 Slim and 2 Bio Cleanse	2 Bio Cleanse	1 ProBio5
28	1 Slim and 2 Bio Cleanse	2 Bio Cleanse	2 ProBio5
28	1 Slim and 2 Bio Cleanse	2 Bio Cleanse	2 ProBio5
30	1 Slim and 2 Bio Cleanse	2 Bio Cleanse	2 ProBio5
31	1 Slim and 2 Bio Cleanse	2 Bio Cleanse	2 ProBio5
32	1 Slim and 2 Bio Cleanse	2 Bio Cleanse	3 ProBio5

DAY	A.M. BEFORE BREAKFAST	P.M. BEFORE DINNER	P.M BEFORE BEDTIME
33	1 Slim and 2 Bio Cleanse	2 Bio Cleanse	3 ProBio5
34	1 Slim and 2 Bio Cleanse	2 Bio Cleanse	3 ProBio5
35	1 Slim and 2 Bio Cleanse	2 Bio Cleanse	3 ProBio5
36	1 Slim and 2 Bio Cleanse	2 Bio Cleanse	4 ProBio5
37	1 Slim and 2 Bio Cleanse	2 Bio Cleanse	4 ProBio5
38	1 Slim and 2 Bio Cleanse	2 Bio Cleanse	4 ProBio5
39	1 Slim and 2 Bio Cleanse	2 Bio Cleanse	4 ProBio5
40	1 Slim and 2 Bio Cleanse	2 Bio Cleanse	4 ProBio5

Made in the USA
Monee, IL
08 October 2020